I0408271

Kama Sutra

The Next Generation

Serg Desire

@ Copyright 2017. All rights reserved.
All rights Reserved. No part of this publication or the information in it may be quoted from or reproduced in any form by means such as printing, scanning, photocopying or otherwise without prior written permission of the copyright holder.

Disclaimer and Terms of Use: Effort has been made to ensure that the information in this book is accurate and complete, however, the author and the publisher do not warrant the accuracy of the information, text and graphics contained within the book due to the rapidly changing nature of science, research, known and unknown facts and internet. The Author and the publisher do not hold any responsibility for errors, omissions or contrary interpretation of the subject matter herein. This book is presented solely for motivational and informational purposes only.

Table of Contents

Part I: Foreplay

Chapter I: Sex Hygiene

Before heading to the sheets, it's important to remember personal hygiene. Picture this: Your hot date has just invited you to their place and you can sense where the mood is going. Things are getting steamy and slowly their mouth makes its way down, down, down. But wait. When was the last time you really cleaned down there? You don't want to be remembered as the person with gunk in their junk. You want to be remembered as the best night of their lives. Here are some pointers on how to maintain good personal hygiene and keep your vagina/penis sparkling.

Women

Vaginas are a very sensitive part of the body and therefore, don't need much to maintain cleanliness. A common misconception is that it needs to be washed, like the rest of your body, with soap. This is wrong. Soap is actually very drying for sensitive skin and can be responsible for itchiness and uncomfort. The vagina only really needs to be washed with warm water to keep it clean. If you decide you want to use soap, make sure it's a plain unscented brand. Other than that there are naturally occurring bacteria that help clean your vagina for you. Your pubic hair also plays a part in your vagina's cleanliness. Shaving or trimming makes it harder for bacteria to grow and live in that area. If you choose to go au natural, make sure to wash that area well as bacterial buildup in that area can also create a bad odor.

What you wear also has an effect on what goes on down there. The vagina needs the right amount of moisture to create the bacteria that keep you clean. If your underwear is too tight it can either cause dryness or too much moisture. If it's too dry, itchiness and rashes can occur that will make you feel very uncomfortable. But if it's too moist, bacterial buildup can occur that can also cause rashes and a strange odor. The best pair of underwear is something made of cotton that is the right fit for your vagina to breath.

Food also plays a part in creating good bacteria and certain foods can make your vaginal juices smell and taste better. Foods, like plain yogurt, contain live cultures of bacteria that aid the bacteria in your vagina. It can also give your vagina a good taste. Many other fruits such as oranges, mangoes and pineapples can give your vagina a good smell and sweeter taste. Really any fruits that have high amounts of natural sugar can have a positive effect on your vaginal juices. At the same time, foods that are highly processed or very strong tastes can make your vagina smell and taste bad. These foods include: onions; garlic; coffee; etc.

Men
Penises are much the same as vaginas and require the same amount of care and cleaning. However, there are two different kinds of penises: circumcised and uncircumcised. Those with uncircumcised penises require a little more attention because of the hood of skin that covers the tip. Here are some pointers on how to keep your penis clean and fresh.

Like vaginas, penises are very sensitive and must be washed with a mild soap. However, if you choose not to use soap, warm water is just as effective. Just make sure to rub all over and under the foreskin, especially if you are uncircumcised. On both types of penises, any part of the foreskin that creates a fold is a place for bacteria to build up. A build up of "smegma" can also occur. Smegma is a natural lubricant that the head of your penis creates. For those that are uncircumcised, if you don't clean under your foreskin, smegma will start to build up which can cause bad odor, itchiness and even infection. When washing also pay attention to the shaft and the testicles. The area between the testicles and the bottom of the shaft creates a lot of moisture this is the perfect breeding ground for bad bacteria. When you're done cleaning, dry your penis and testicles thoroughly with a soft towel. Try to avoid using body powders on this area as it can dry your penis and testicles too much and cause a rash and/or itchiness.

Some men are notorious for wearing the same outfit for a week. When it comes to underwear: DON'T DO THIS! After washing your penis make sure to put on a clean pair of underwear. (And flipping it inside out doesn't count.) The type of underwear you choose is up to you. Some like the tightness of briefs while others like the free flow of boxers. Just make sure the underwear you choose isn't too tight. Not only is it uncomfortable but constricting your testicles could cause problems for your sperm. If you choose to go commando, you'll have to pay more attention when you clean yourself. Little bits of cloth from your pants can get stuck to the tip or under the foreskin. No matter what you choose during the day, when you sleep it's a good idea to not wear any underwear. This gives your penis and testicles a chance to breath. All the sweat from your clothes that's built up during the day gets a chance to air out, which helps prevent infection.

Food can make a penis taste better and even help with erections. Fresh fruits and vegetables are great for helping penises smell and taste good. But unlike women, things such as coffee and spicy food are great for a man's libido. Coffee is a great way to prevent erectile dysfunction because the caffeine helps stimulate blood flow to the penis. Spicy food is shown to increase testosterone levels and in turn increase the size of an erect penis. As long as you eat healthy, well-made foods you should be fine. Stay away from the highly processed, fake foods. And make sure not to drink too much booze on your date. It desensitizes you and makes your reaction time slower. Meaning it'll be harder for you to "get it up" and a very unsatisfied date.

Sexual Hygiene
You've kept up a routine and you're feeling fresher than ever, but what about your partner? If you're going to have

sex with someone you haven't known for long, it's important to keep yourself protected. The most important thing to remember is: ALWAYS use a condom. Unless you've been with your partner for a significant amount of time and know their sexual history you should always use a condom. It may be uncomfortable and not feel as good but it will protect you from the truly horrendous STI's that are out there.

If, for some reason, you didn't use a condom during one of your sexual adventures, you need to go for a checkup. And even if you use protection, it's advisable that you go for regular checkups (at least once a year) to make sure that everything is in working order. If you are in a long term relationship, it's also a good idea to check each other for any signs of infection or abnormalities such as rashes or tearing.

When having sex, it's important that both partners are thoroughly warmed up. This helps create natural lube that makes penetration easier and safer. If the woman is having trouble getting wet (which can be caused by many reasons) having lube on hand is very useful. Don't force penetration if the woman isn't lubricated. This can cause tearing of both, the vaginal wall and the foreskin. Lube is also important if you are choosing to have anal sex, since the anus doesn't produce any natural lubrication. After having sex, both partners should wash their genitals to clean off any fluids that could build up and cause bacterial infection.

If you follow these tips and build a good routine, you and your partner will stay healthy, happy and be ready to embark on your sexual adventure.

Chapter 2: Oral Sex

Blowjobs

A blowjob is much more than sucking a penis up and down. If you're tired of the same routine or you want to surprise your man with something new, here are 20 different ways to fellatio your partner.

The Standard

This is your everyday blowjob. But just because it's the "everyday blowjob" doesn't mean it can't be something special. The beauty about the standard blowjob is that you don't have to do anything fancy. All you really need to do is take your time. Show your man you want to be down there and that you enjoy it just as much as him.

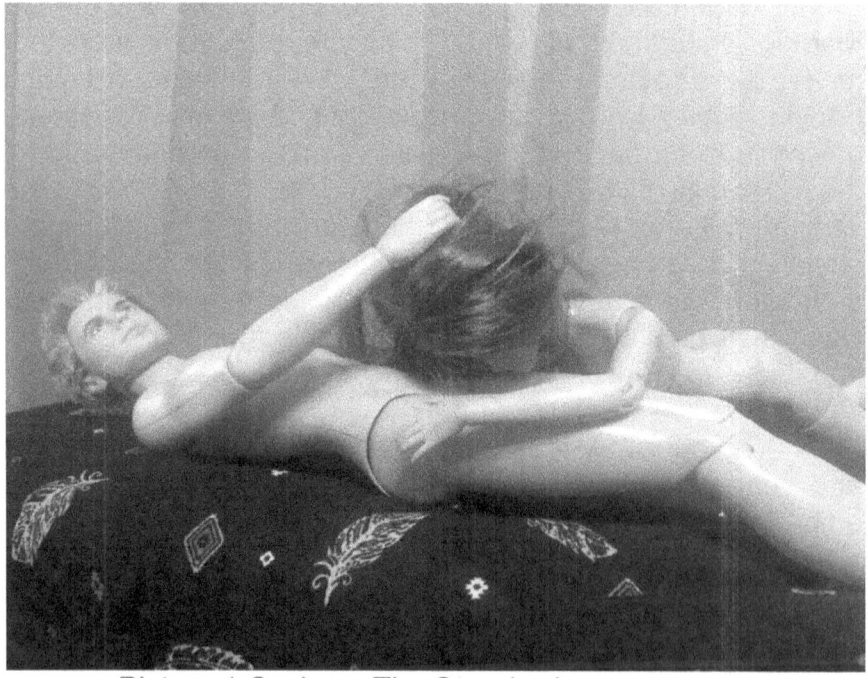

Picture 1 Oral sex The Standard

Start by having your man lie on his back while you're between his legs. Starting from the base of his penis like all the way to the tip of his penis. Then take the tip into your mouth and slowly work your way back down (as far as you feel comfortable). If your man is uncircumcised either gently pull down his foreskin with your hand or push it down with your lips as you lower your head. Continue moving up and down in a steady rhythm while gently sucking on his penis. Start moving faster and faster, all the while keeping a constant rhythm, until you start to feel him getting ready to cum. When you feel that he's about to come don't increase your speed. Keep moving your head up and down at your current speed but begin to suck him a bit stronger. In a matter of seconds, you'll have him in the palm of your hand. Or should I say mouth?

The Lollipop

This move is for girls who a bit more timid. It probably won't lead your man to orgasm but if your goal is to get him revved up, this is the perfect technique.

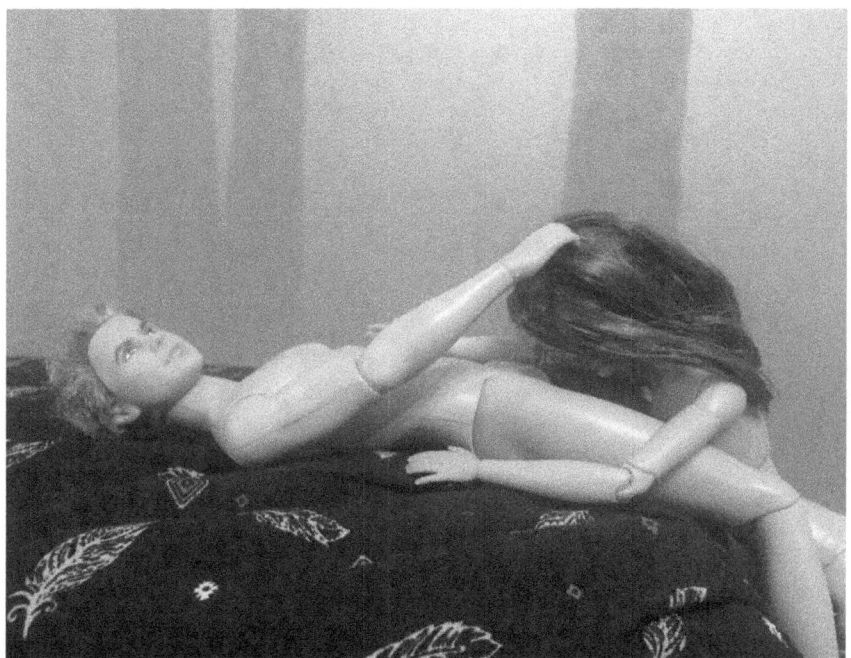

Picture 2 Oral sex The The Lollipop

Start by letting your man get comfortable and then position yourself between his legs. Starting from the base, slowly lick all the way to the tip of his penis. Once at the tip (if he is uncircumcised gently pull his foreskin down with your hand until the tip of his penis is completely uncovered) gently rub your tongue around the tip of his penis. Vary your tongue technique for optimal pleasure. You can lightly flick the tip with the point of your tongue, swirl it completely around the tip, gently press the hole at the top with the point of your tongue and/or lick up and down the entirety of his member. The general idea of this technique is to be playful and teasing so get creative with it.

Double Trouble

Combination is key here. This move requires you to use both your mouth and your hand. By applying different pressures and varying the movement between your mouth and hands you'll have him writhing with pleasure.

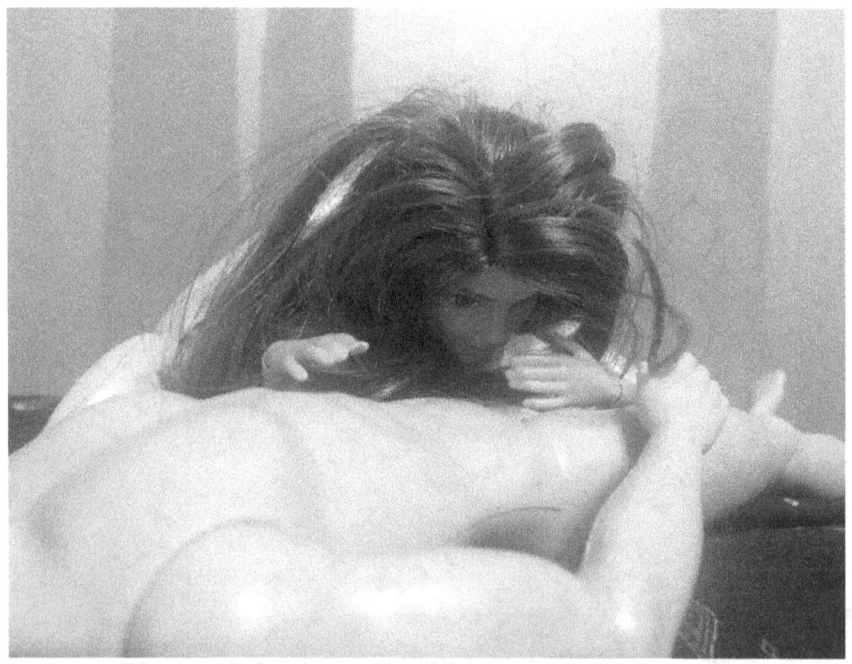

Picture 3 Oral sex Double Trouble

Begin by placing your hand at the bottom of his shaft and slowly stroking up and down. After a few moments of this, slowly lower your mouth around the tip of his penis and gently suck. Continue stroking the length of his penis as you only suck and/or lick the tip. Lower your head until half of his penis is in your mouth and the other half is being stroked by your hand. If you want to change things up, start swirling your tongue around his penis in one direction while you gently twist your hand around his shaft in the other direction. Another trick is to pretend to be pushing more of his penis into your mouth. To do this keep sucking up and down in one area while you gently pull up from the bottom of his penis. As you do this, increase the strength of your sucking. The main point of this move is variation. Create different combinations with your hands and mouth to arouse different sensations.

The Magician or The Prisoner
The exact opposite of double trouble. This move can be done two ways and it all depends on how adventurous you are. Either option is a little more advanced because it requires a lot of neck strength and good breathing techniques.

The first option is called The Magician. First he sees your hands, then he doesn't. While you're on your knees start out by doing The Lollipop or The Standard. If you're new to this and your hands are on his penis put them on his thighs while you continue moving your head up and down. If you're more experienced or you're feeling comfortable, remove your hands from his body all together. Place them on your thighs and continue sucking his penis as you move your head up and down. This option is the easier version because if you're feeling tired or running out of breath you can put your hands back on his body or penis.

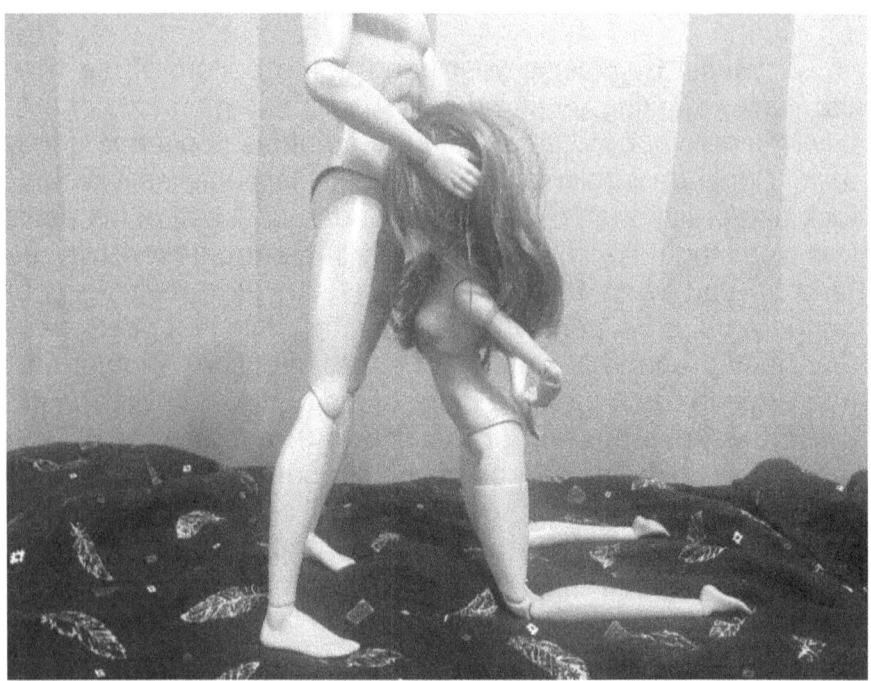
Picture 4 Oral sex The Prisoner

The Prisoner is the more advanced option. This move requires your hands to be tied or handcuffed behind your back. Make sure you and your partner are both in comfortable positions. It is also important that you and your partner have good bodily communication so they can sense your limits and not go past. Once your hands are behind your back, lower your mouth around his penis and combine techniques for The Lollipop and The Standard. Remember to pace yourself. This position is tiring for the neck and mouth so if you want to last, start out slow and work your way up to a speed that's comfortable for you. If you start feeling tired or uncomfortable let your partner know and stop. The last thing you want to do is pass out.

The Explorer
For those who have a partner with foreskin, this is the move for you. Men with foreskin have more sensitive penises. This doesn't mean that you can skimp on technique. It just

means everything you do is felt stronger. Use the foreskin to your advantage.

Start out by licking all around the base of his penis and the length of his shaft. When you get to the tip don't immediately pull his foreskin down. Instead, stick your tongue into his foreskin and slowly move it around the tip of his penis. The sensation will be doubled because he'll feel it on the inside of his foreskin (somewhere that normally doesn't get stimulated) and on the tip of his penis. Then, place your mouth around the very tip of his foreskin and lower your head. This will roll his foreskin down and put the tip of his penis straight into your mouth. This move is best done as one fluid movement. This means to continue inserting his penis into your mouth even once the tip of his penis has been completely revealed.

The Prayer
This move allows for a bigger range of motion. Have your man sit at the edge of the bed or on a chair.

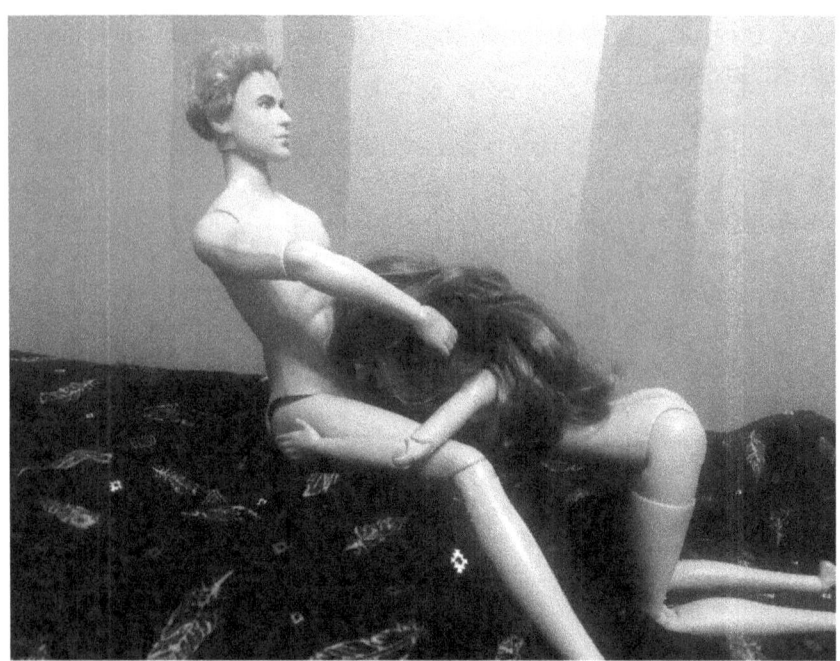

Picture 5 Oral sex The Prayer

Position yourself, kneeling between his legs. The beauty of this move is that you can incorporate any of the other techniques into this position. This technique is mostly about positioning. Because his penis is level with your face you are able to do more without straining yourself as much.

The Pearly White

Some men like this move and others hate it, so make sure your man is ok with you using teeth before you attempt this.

Incorporate this with other techniques that you wish to use. While you are sucking his penis very lightly scrape your teeth across the tip of his penis. Don't do this more than once at a time because it can make his penis very sore. You can also scrape your teeth across the length of his shaft as you're moving your head up. The further down you are the harder you can scrape as it's less sensitive than the tip. But again it's also up to your man's preferences. When you are more towards the bottom of his shaft, stop moving and slowly bite down until you feel him tense. Then release and resume sucking up and down.

Ice Ice Baby

Men really enjoy this move. The sensation between hot and cold is very stimulating for their penis.

Choose between either an ice cube or a mint. (A mint is preferable if you're new to this move.) If you choose an ice cube, make sure it's small enough so you can also put his penis in your mouth comfortably. Put the mint or ice in your mouth and swirl it around so all parts of your mouth absorb the cold. Then slowly put his penis in your mouth. In the beginning try to keep the mint or ice from directly touching his penis (the shock of cold could cause him to loose wood). As you move your mouth up and down, alternate pressing the mint or ice against his penis and removing it. You can also swirl it around the whole of his penis with your tongue. Just remember to remove the mint or ice from his penis occasionally so he can feel the alternation sensations of hot and cold

The Anaconda

The Standard with a little extra. This is a more advanced move and requires you to loosen up your throat. Don't attempt this move if you have a very sensitive gag reflex. You don't want to be throwing up all over your man. You can practice this move when you brush your teeth or when you eat a banana. Try inserting, whatever you choose, further and further into the back of your mouth and into the opening of your throat. What you really want to do here is relax your throat muscles so that his penis can slide down and hit the very back of your throat. When you think you're ready try it with his penis. It's best if you start with The Standard or The Lollipop so that you can warm up your mouth and throat. (Don't immediately stick his penis down your throat.) When you're warmed up, slowly start sliding your mouth down his penis as far as you can. You're going to meet resistance at some point (this is your gag reflex). When this happens stop for a second and let your throat get use to the sensation. Then continue moving down as far as you feel comfortable. If you make a gagging noise (which is most likely going to happen) don't be embarrassed. Men actually love this noise!

The Sweet Surprise

This move is really fun and you can get really creative with it. You will be using food so it's advisable to put some towels down or to do it on a surface that can be easily cleaned. The best food for this move is anything liquid and sweet. This can be anything from honey, to whipped cream. The point is to pick something that you really enjoy eating.

When you've chosen your "secret ingredient," dribble it onto his penis. Dribbling is the best method for application because it creates a unique sensation on his penis. Try not to use too much of your food because you'll have to lick it all off by the end. Once the food is on his penis begin by lightly licking it off. Then proceed to nibbling the tip and eventually move to "eating" his whole member. The sweet stuff is supposed to encourage you to really "go at it" with his penis. Not only does it feel great for him but he also gets to watch you enjoy licking him.

Wet N' Wild

This move requires a lot of saliva. Start out with a simple sucking technique to warm yourself up and get your saliva flowing. When you start feeling like there is a lot of saliva in your mouth, simply keep going. Don't try to swallow the excess, just let it run down his penis. It may feel like there's a lot of water building up around his crotch but that's the point. The excess wetness makes your sucking technique feel extra slippery and can even mimic what sex feels like. For an added bonus: if you're feeling brave try spitting on his penis. Men love this extra dirty move. When you remove your mouth from his penis try letting the saliva dribble from your mouth onto your chin or his crotch. It's a very hot move that'll really get his engine revving.

The Baller

When it comes to fellatio the testicles are often neglected, but when done properly they can provide a great amount of stimulation for a man and even help him orgasm. It's important to remember that men's testicles are very, very sensitive so you must be extra careful when handling them.

As you are sucking his penis, start caressing his testicles with your hand. Lightly squeeze them and move them around, almost like you're massaging them. Then, remove your mouth from around his penis and start licking his testicles. Swirling your tongue around them has a nice sensation but simply licking them up and down is also good. If you feel comfortable, lightly suck one of his testicles into your mouth. Gently tug with your mouth and swirl your tongue around it. Repeat this with the other one. You can also put both of them into your mouth and swirl your tongue in an 8 pattern. Remember never to suck them hard or use your teeth.

If you are more advanced you can try putting his penis and his testicles in mouth all at once. You will need to be able to do The Anaconda for this more advanced move. Start by sucking his penis. Move as far down as you can. The closer you are to the bottom of his shaft the easier this will be. Once you're towards the bottom of his shaft, open your mouth as wide as possible and gently stick his testicles into your mouth. You won't be able to move your head up and down once they're in your mouth but you can gently suck on both his penis and testicles at the same time. You can also try swirling your tongue around in an 8 pattern.

Risky Business

If you're extremely adventurous, then this is for you. This move isn't so much about technique as it is location. Where you choose to give your man a blowjob is the thrill of this move. The idea is to give him a blowjob in a public place or a place where you could easily get caught. You will need to get creative and be fast. So this move doesn't really rely on technique as much. The best places for this move are: a bathroom; in the park/forest behind a tree; an airplane; a movie theater; and a taxi. But you can also choose where you want to do it. Spontaneity is key. Don't tell your man what you're about to do. Just grab him, bring him to a secluded location and start going down on him. It's almost guaranteed that he will love it.

Tip: If you're doing it where there are other people close by, such as an airplane, pretend to be sleeping on his lap. Cover his penis and your mouth with a blanket and try not to move your head as much. This means you'll need to get creative with tongue movements and mouth pressure, but the tension from the situation should help elevate the sensations that he's feeling.

Dinner for Two
Both of you get to enjoy this move. It's the infamous 69. There are a number of ways for you and your partner to position yourselves, but there's not special technique employed to actually fellatio him. The most common positions are side to side or one on top of the other. Either you or your partner turn around so the both your faces are in front of each others genitals. This position is optimal for doing all the techniques listed, especially The Baller. The main idea of this position is that both of you get pleasure at the same time. Make sure not to get too caught up with what he's doing and forget to please him. This position is all about balance.

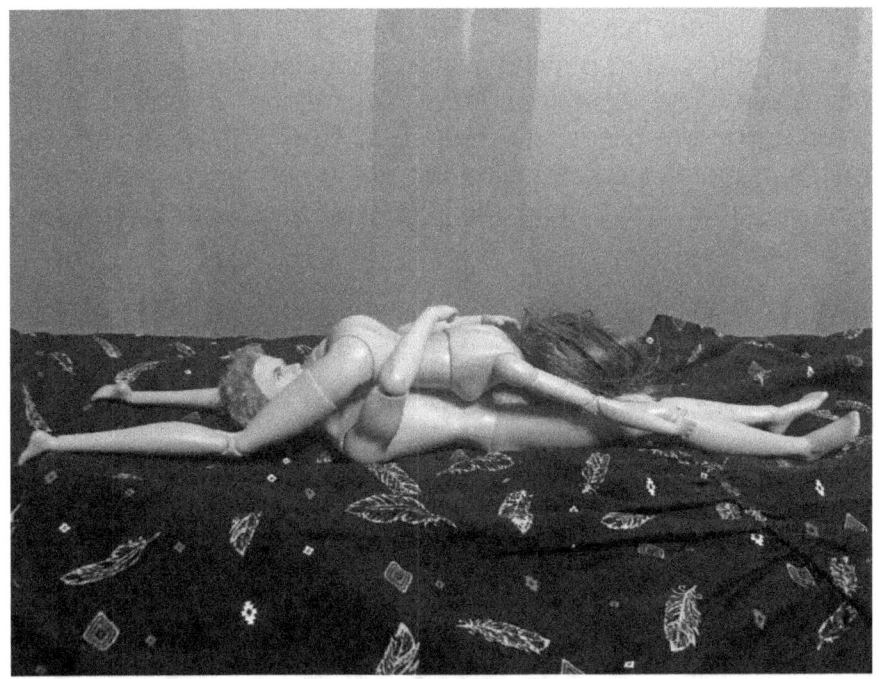

Picture 6 Oral sex Dinner for Two

Tip: If he's on top make sure you can communicate to him your airflow. It's easy for him to forget what he's doing and suffocate you with his weight. Have some way to let him know that he needs to stop.

The Back Door

For this move, you should make sure your partner knows what's going to happen and is onboard with it. If you have long nails it's advisable that you either, don't do this move or your trim them. You can choose any variation of blowjob and do it for however long you want. While you are sucking his penis, take your index or middle finger and press it up against his butthole. Don't' immediately stick it in. The anus is very tight and is also not naturally lubricated. You should either lick your finger or apply some lube to it before you insert it. While your finger is pressed up to his butthole start massaging and inserting it in slowly. Let his anus get use to the feeling of something going inside it. If you've managed to get your whole finger into his butthole and he's gotten use to the sensation, start moving it in and out slowly as your sucking his penis. The combination of sensations is going to be strange for him but it should end up feeling really good. The man's g-spot is located inside the anus, behind the prostate. If you can manage to find this, he will have one of the best orgasms of his life.

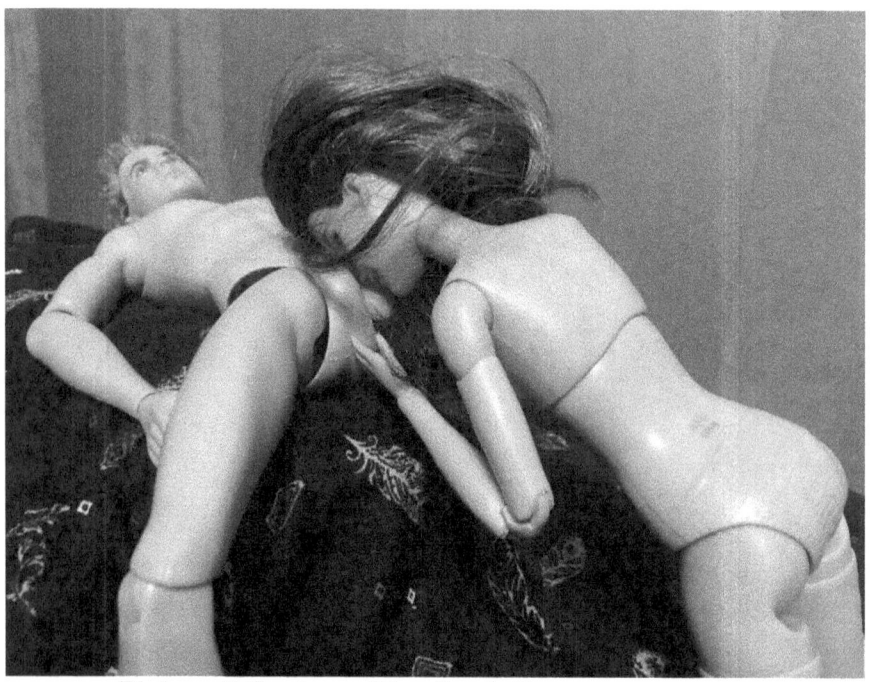

Picture 7 Oral sex The Back Door

The Head Fuck

This move requires some initiative from your man. Position yourselves so that he is standing and you are kneeling in front of him. You can use any technique for this move except for The Baller and The Pearly Whites. This move is can be pretty aggressive so make sure not to do anything too hard with your mouth.

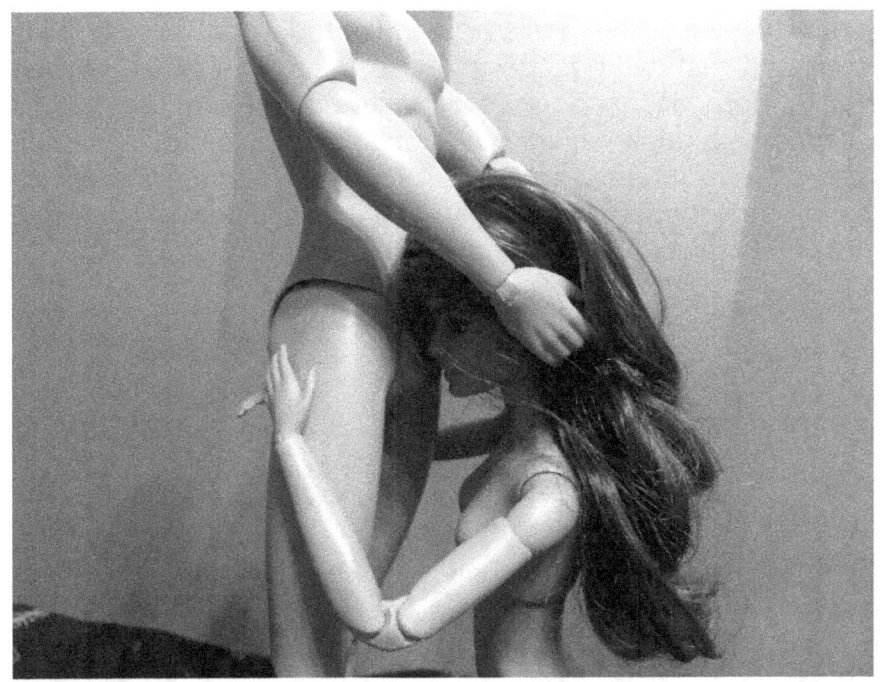

Picture 8 Oral sex The Head Fuck

As you are sucking his penis have him put his hands on your head or in your hair and let him control your movement. Relax your neck so that he can take control of you without meeting resistance. Again, this is why your jaw should stay relaxed so you don't accidentally scrape his penis too hard. It's important to listen to what his hands are telling you to do. He can communicate a lot, such as speed and how hard you should be sucking. This doesn't mean that you can't throw in some moves of your own. Try alternating between sucking and using your tongue. He can't control what your tongue does so use it to your advantage.

The Porno

One of the more advanced moves and is the perfect position for The Anaconda. Lay on your back, on a raised surface while he stands near your head. Rest the bottom of your head on the edge of the surface so that your head dangles over. Open your mouth wide, relax your neck and let him slowly insert his penis. Have his stop when he's half way so your throat can get use to the feeling and pressure. When you're more loosened up let him take control and thrust at his own speed. Make sure you don't just lie there. Alternate sucking pressures and use your tongue. This position allows him to go very deep in your throat, so don't attempt it if you're not comfortable with The Anaconda.

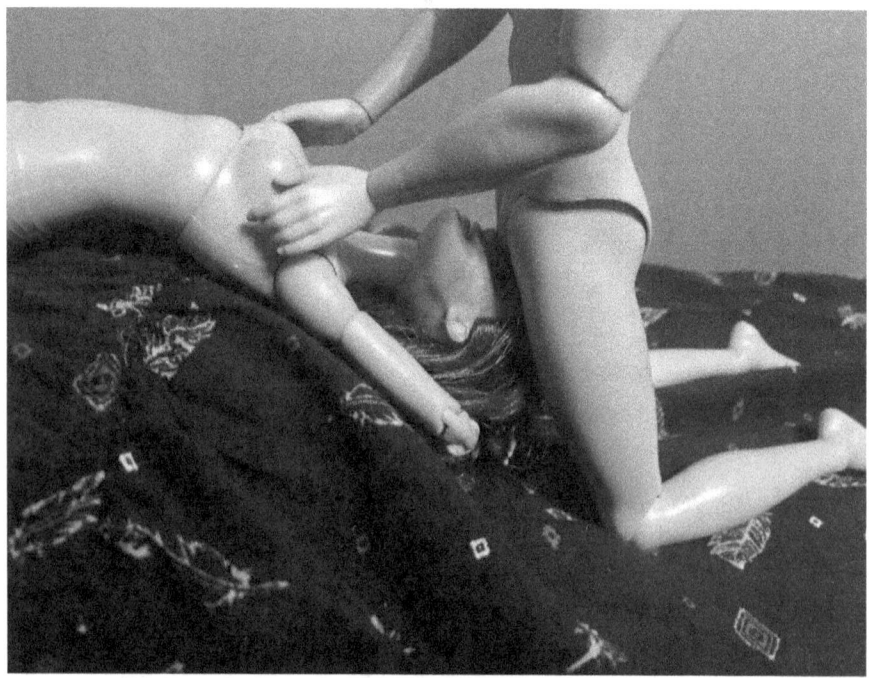

Picture 9 Oral sex The Porno

Another added bonus of this move is that he can see his penis pressing into your throat which is a big turn on for him.

The Dominator

This move is a more comfortable version of The Porno. For this technique you're going to lie on your back. Have your partner put his knees on either side of your head so that his penis is close to or above your mouth. To make this more comfortable, prop your head up with a pillow so that you don't strain your neck. If you need to, lift your head up so that you can put his penis in your mouth. You can use any of the techniques listed her to give him a fantastic blowjob. This position also allows him to take control and thrust into your mouth at his own speed. Try combining this move with The Baller for an ultimate experience.

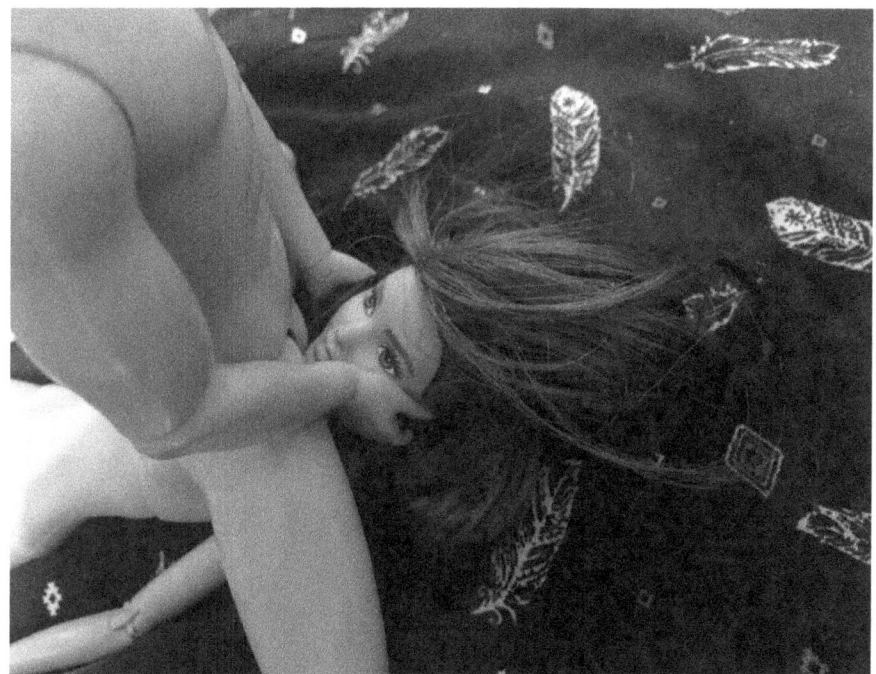

Picture 10 Oral sex The Dominator

The Handstand

Only attempt this move if you can do a perfect handstand and have strong arm muscles. (If you do want to attempt this move and you don't have good balance, try using a wall for support.) This move isn't meant to last too long because you might pass out, but it is a really creative way to spice things up with your foreplay. It's basically a combination of The Porno and Dinner for Two.

Position yourself by getting into a handstand. Make sure you're stable and as comfortable as you can get. It also helps if your man holds your legs or you butt for stability. Your face should be level with his penis. If not, he may have to squat a little, but if you're too short this move isn't for you. Once your mouth is level with his penis, insert it and start your blowjob techniques. You probably won't be able to do anything fancy because your concentration will be on balancing but your partner can help you by thrusting and doing much of the movement. Remember not to stay in this position for too long or you might pass out. When you're finished, come out of the position slowly. All the blood has rushed to your head and you've been deprived of oxygen so you'll probably be slightly lightheaded and dizzy.

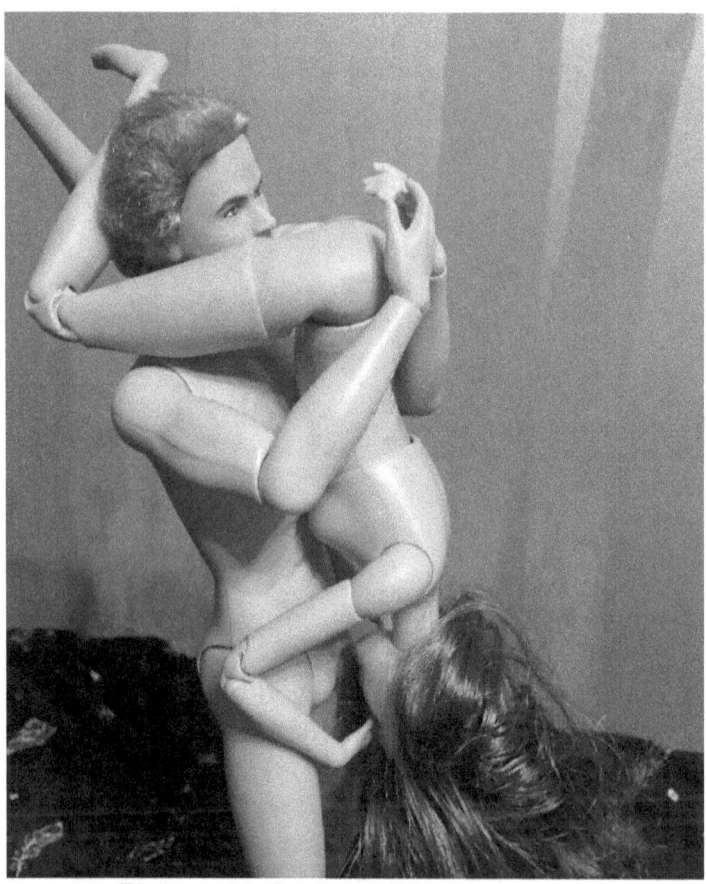

Picture 11 Oral sex The Handstand

The Backbend

Only attempt this move if both of you are really flexible and strong. This position is the most advanced, next to The Handstand. If you're aim is to be really adventurous and mimic a porno, this is the move for you.

Start by getting into a backbend and then have your partner position himself so that his penis is near your mouth. You may have to lift your neck a little so that he can insert his penis comfortably in your mouth. This move is strenuous on the back and neck so make sure you don't clench your jaw or your throat as this could end up hurting both of you. When his penis is in your mouth have him start thrusting. He will have to be in charge of movement. Because of the angle you are in, he should be able to thrust his penis deep into your throat. Make sure to alternate sucking pressure and tongue movement as much as you can. Stay in this position as long as both of you feel comfortable. Over exerting yourself can cause injury to either of you.

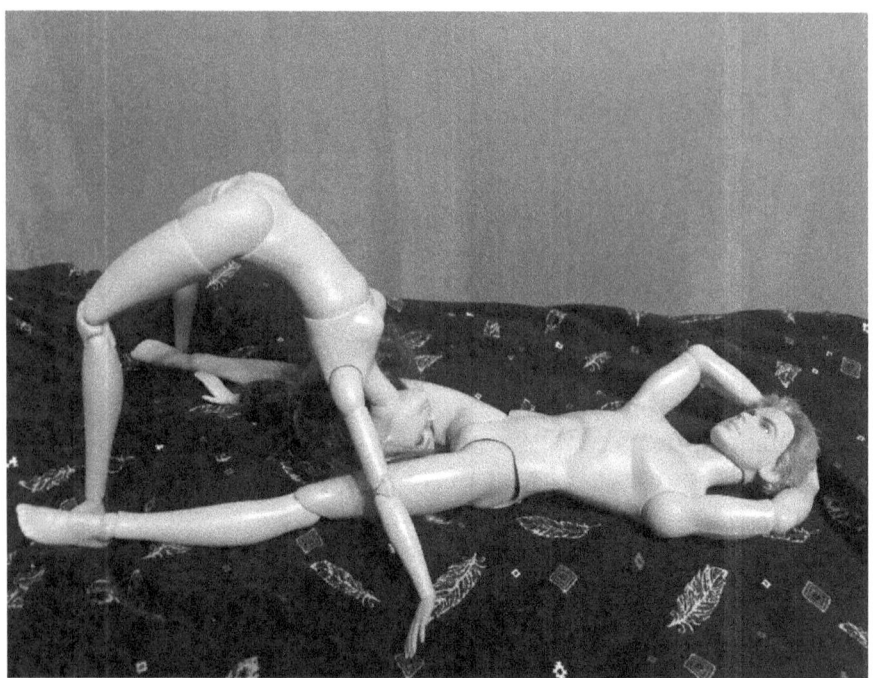
Picture 12 Oral sex The Backbend

Remember that variety and enthusiasm are key to any good blowjob. You don't have to stick with just one technique. Mix it up and no matter which you choose don't forget that communication is key. What works for some men might be a turn off for others. Read his body language and if you're ever in doubt, ask. Men like knowing that what you really want to do, is please them.

Cunnilingus

Let's face it. When it comes to going down on a woman, most men are clueless. Women tend to have more needs than men and cunnilingus begins well before you actually go down on your woman. Don't immediately go straight to eating her out. Take time to warm her up through kissing and touching her body. When she's loosened up and gotten her juices flowing, then start to make your way down. If you're feeling stuck on what to do here are 18 different ways to pleasure your woman.

The Standard

This is the equivalent of the man's standard blowjob and is the basic foundation of any other techniques.

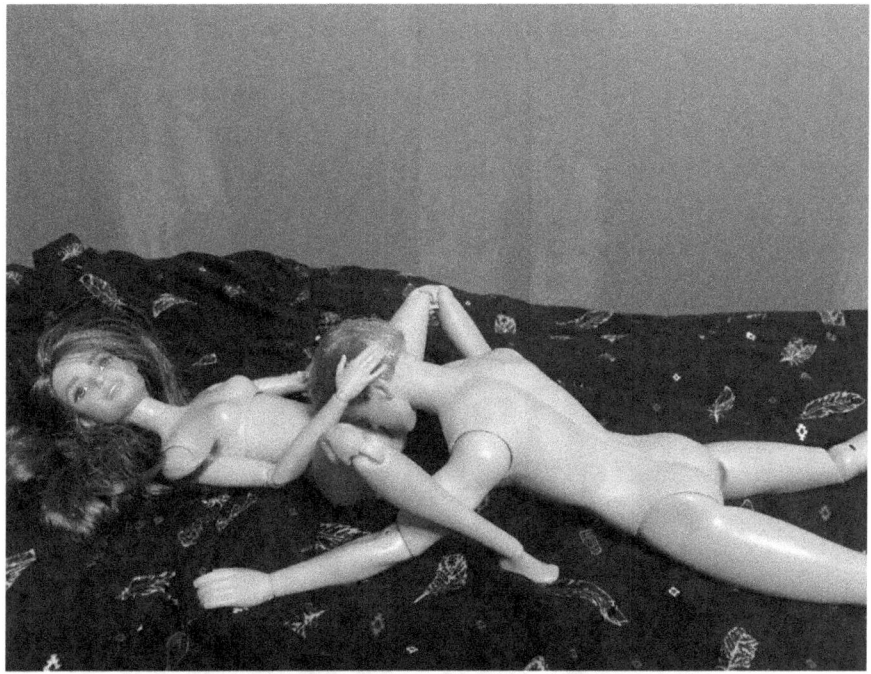

Picture 13 Cunnilingus The Standard

Slowly kiss her body as you make your way down. When you've positioned yourself between her legs, part the lips of her vagina with your fingers and lower your mouth onto it. Start by licking all around, getting her lubed up. Use your tongue to flick her clit several times. (This is the most sensitive part of the vagina.) You can even insert your tongue into her vaginal opening. Swirl it around and/or thrust it in and out. If your aim is to make her orgasm, it may take several minutes to reach that point. Don't be discouraged. Alternate movements so your tongue doesn't get worn out. Several techniques listed below will help give your tongue a break. If you are just trying to get her lubed up for sex, make sure you spend enough time pleasuring her before you stop.

The Surprise

This pose is like The Standard but from behind. Have your woman lie on her stomach and place a pillow underneath her pelvis. This will help put her in a position that gives you a better angle. Spread her legs but make sure the pillow is still supporting her and pushing her butt slightly up. (Long body pillows are the best support but you can also use several pillows together.) You can also place your hands on the front side of her hips and push up so that you have more room for variation. Only attempt this move if you are comfortable with her anus near your face. Once you're both in position begin going down on her. Your mouth and nose will be buried in her crotch so make sure you take breaks for breath.

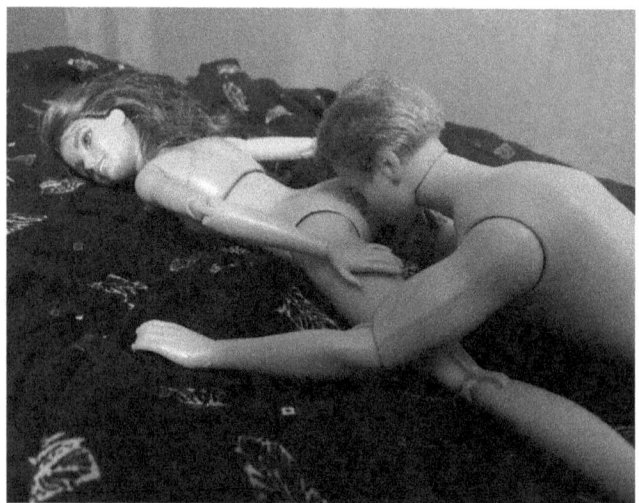

Picture 14 Cunnilingus The Surprise

The Window Washer

The Window Washer is a great move if your woman is a little more adventurous. Choose a window that is easily accessible and relatively big. The best would be a sliding glass door or a large window in your living room or bedroom. After you've warmed her up and stripped her down get her to stand up and face the window. Have her lean at a 45-degree angle so that her breasts are pressed against the surface and her butt sticks out. Position yourself in front of her and spread her legs. Then start licking her as you normally would. Alternatively, you can have her stick her butt out further and go down on her from behind. (This position will be explained later.) The idea of this pose is to heighten sensations through the fear of being caught. This pose increases adrenaline and makes the body more sensitive to strong sensations.

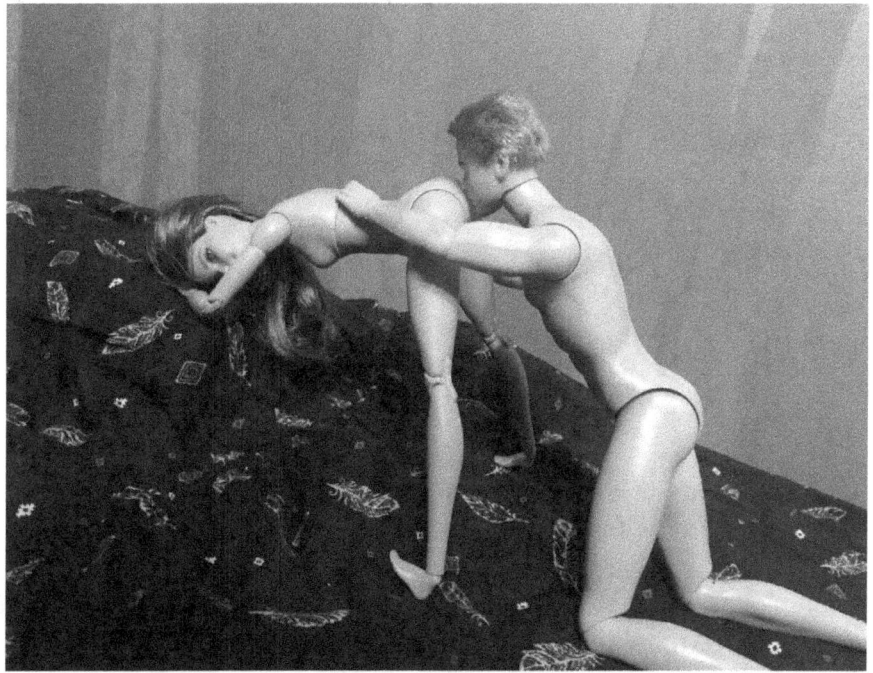

Picture 15 Cunnilingus The Window Washer

Dinner for Two

This move is the same as Dinner for Two in the previous section on blowjobs. To recapitulate, turn yourself so that your face is near her vagina and her face is near your penis. You can do this while lying side to side or one on top of the other. When you both are comfortable, place your mouth on her vagina and start licking and/or sucking. Remember to pay touch the to whole vagina but give special attention to the clitoris and the vaginal opening.

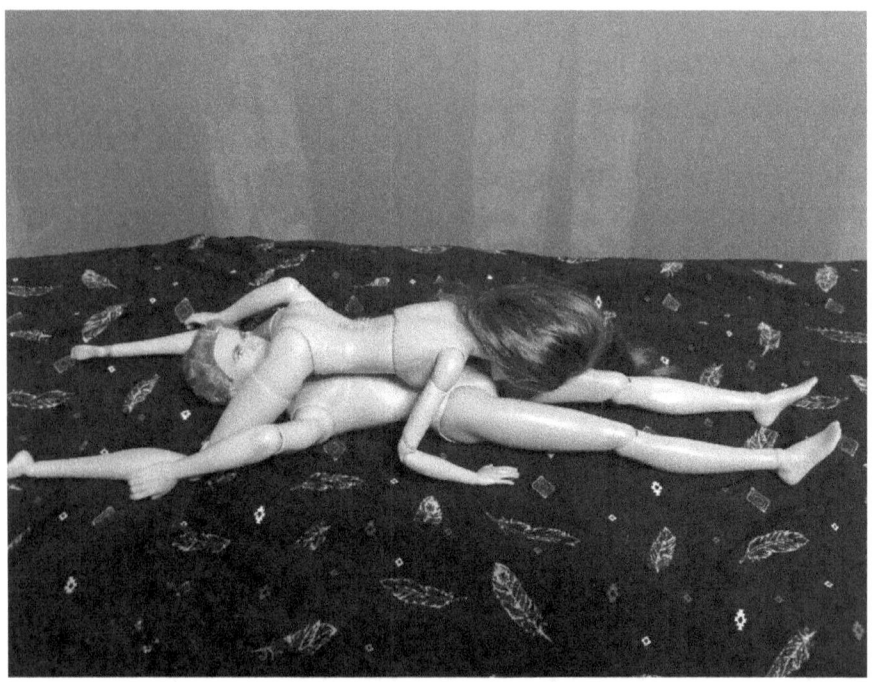
Picture 16 Cunnilingus Dinner for Two

A variation of this move would be to place your head between her thighs while you are in a side to side position. Then have gently squeeze them together as you eat her out. This allows her to relax and feel the sensations more deeply. It can also be quite stimulating for yourself.

The Downward Dog
A sexy variation of the yoga pose. Have your woman get into the position of downward dog. (Start on all fours and then push your knees away from the floor so your feet come closer to the floor and your head remains near the ground.) When she is comfortable, help her spread her legs far enough apart that you can situate yourself between them. Because of this position her vagina should be up in the air and easily accessible. Spread her lips and begin gently licking her. This pose makes her vagina very vulnerable and therefore increases its sensitivity. Make sure not to stay in this position for very long as blood will be rushing to her head and can

cause her to pass out. Depending on how long you stay in this position and if she was able to orgasm, she could be very lightheaded and dizzy so make sure to help her come out of it.

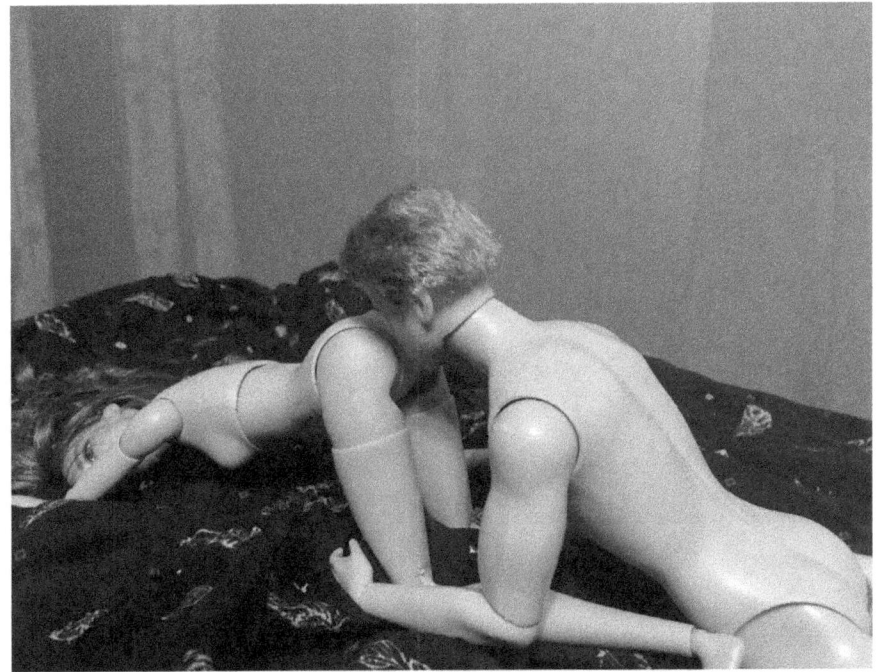

Picture 17 Cunnilingus The Downward Dog

The Boss

The Boss is a great move for women that like to feel in charge and if you like feeling dominated. Begin by having her sit in a chair. She can be naked or clothed. If she chooses to wear clothes make sure it's something easily accessible or removable, such as a skirt. This position is felt best if she can recline in the chair. Place yourself between her legs, part her vagina and proceed with going down on her. You can also put her legs over your shoulder for a better angle.

Tip: Trying throwing in a little role play with this move for maximum effectiveness. Empowerment is a big turn on for women.

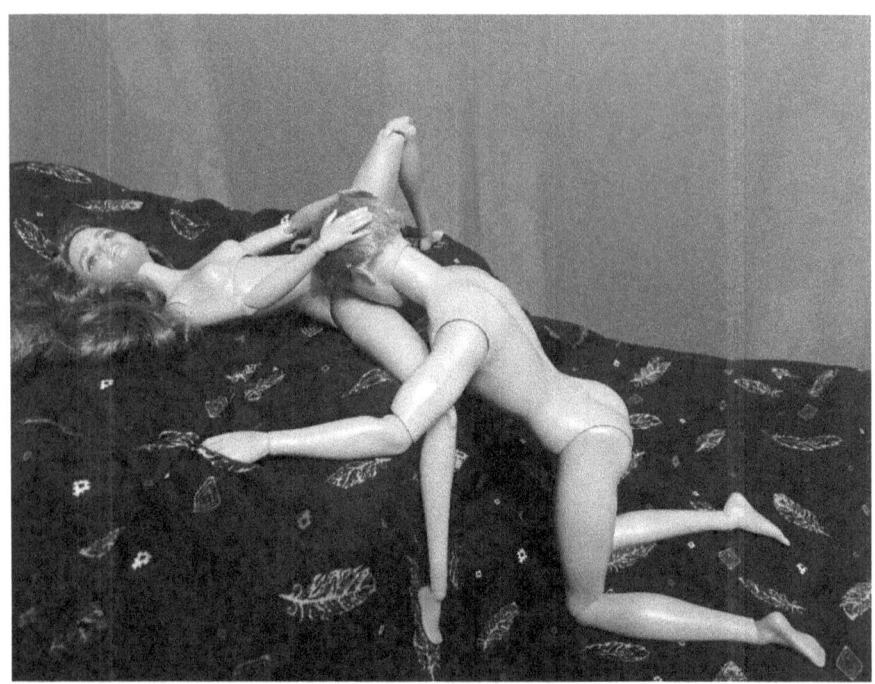

Picture 18 Cunnilingus The Boss

The Chair

This move sounds like the previous one but there's a slight difference. Your face becomes the chair that she sits on. Start by lying on your back, on a comfortable surface. Then have her place her knees on either side of your head so that her vagina is above your mouth. When both of you are ready, let her lower herself on to your open mouth. This move is amazing for her because she can control the pressure on her vagina. Try placing your tongue only on her clit and letting her rub it against you. Make sure you do something with your hands as well. Grab her breasts and massage them or grab/smack her butt for extra effect.

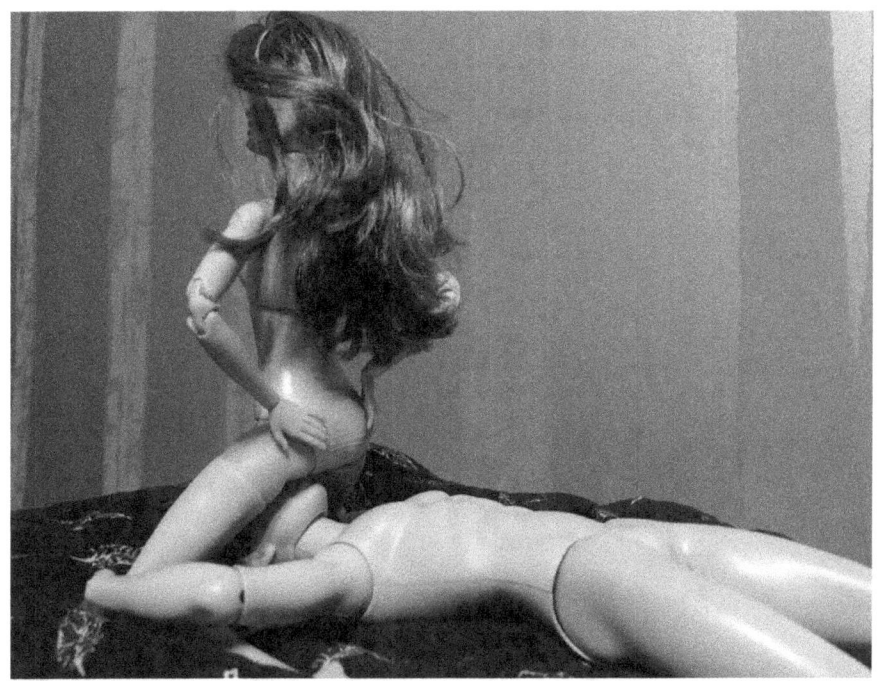

Picture 19 Cunnilingus The Chair

The On the Go

On the Go is a great move for a quickie. This move doesn't require either of you to get undressed. But it's better if your woman is wearing something easily accessible, like a skirt or dress. Make this move spontaneous. When she's getting ready or even when she's about to leave. Press her up against a wall and lower yourself so that you're in front of her vagina. Quickly remove any clothing that's covering it up and begin to eat her out. Use lots of variation and pressure, paying close attention to the clitoris. This move needs to be fast so you need to make her orgasm as quickly as you can. When she orgasms, put her clothes back on and send her on her way!

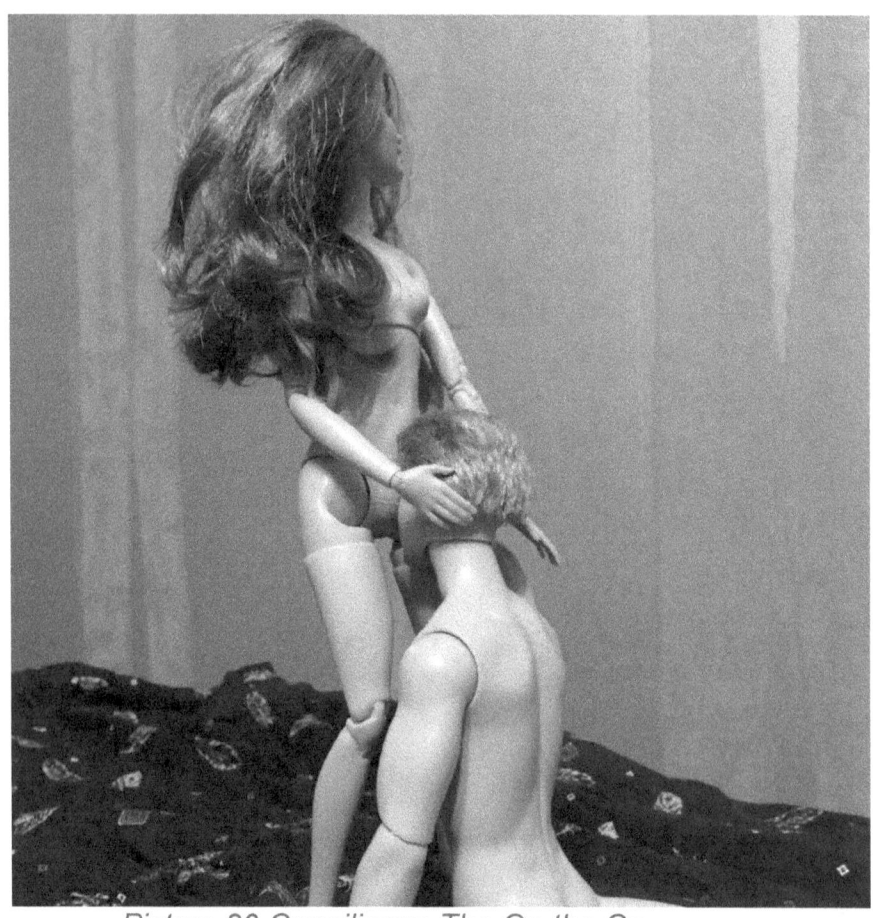

Picture 20 Cunnilingus The On the Go

The Tree Hugger

This position is a more advanced version of The Window Washer because it requires you to be in public. The best place for this move is the forest or the park (somewhere that has trees.) Pull her bottoms off and have her lean her upper torso on a tree for balance. You can either position yourself in front or behind her. Spread her legs and start licking her vagina. Try to get her really riled up, to the point where she's making noise. She's going to try to hold it in which is going to make her feel even more turned on. If you want, you can also make it a quickie since there is the chance you could get caught.

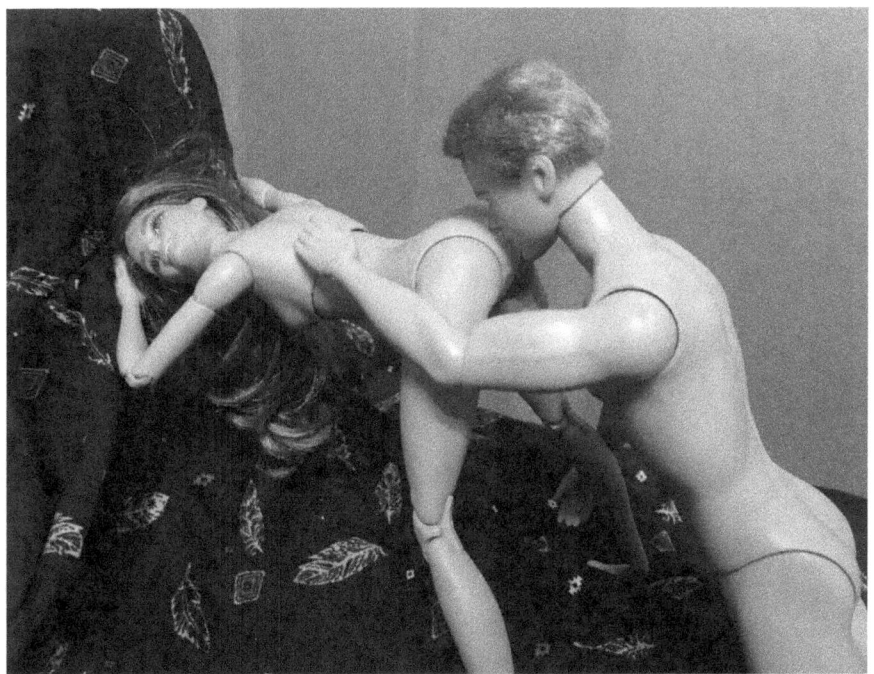

Picture 21 Cunnilingus The Tree Hugger

Tip: If both of you are strong enough and the tree is small enough, have her wrap her arms around it and hold on tight. Then lift her legs off the ground while you eat her out. This move can get pretty tiring for both of you so don't attempt to do it for too long.

The Bad Girl

This pose is a variation of The Surprise. It requires an elevated surface, such as a table. Have her stand so that her legs are pressed up against the elevated surface and then bend her over so that her torso is lying on top of it. Spread her legs and lower your mouth onto her vagina. You can kneel or position a chair between her legs and sit on that. This position also works with her lying on her back with her legs dangling. It is also a great pose for your viewing pleasure.

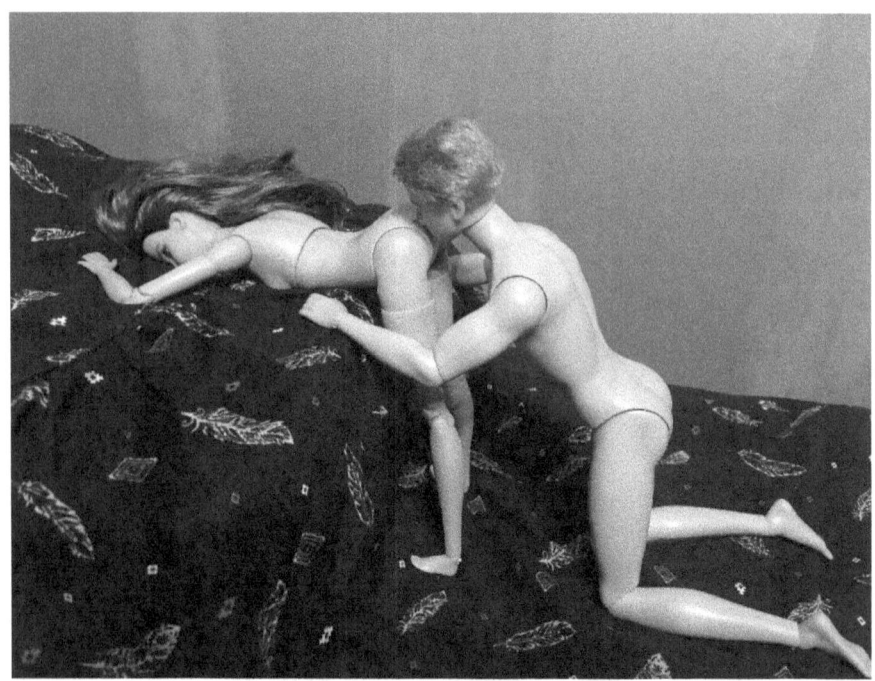

Picture 22 Cunnilingus The Bad Girl

Tip: If you want to get kinkier with this pose you can tie her legs to the table and her hands behind her back. (For more on BDSM see Chapter 3.)

Spread Eagle

For this pose you're going to need a soft rope or cloth to tie her legs. This can be used in combination with The Bad Girl or it can be a separate pose on its own. It best if there's something nearby that you can tie her legs to but if that's not possible you can also tie her hands to her ankles. This will keep her from being able to comfortably close her legs. Make sure the material you use to tie her up is non-irritating and not too tight. When her legs are tied apart, start teasing her with your mouth. This position is best for focusing on sensitive areas and teasing her. She won't be able to stop you so use this opportunity to drive her wild.

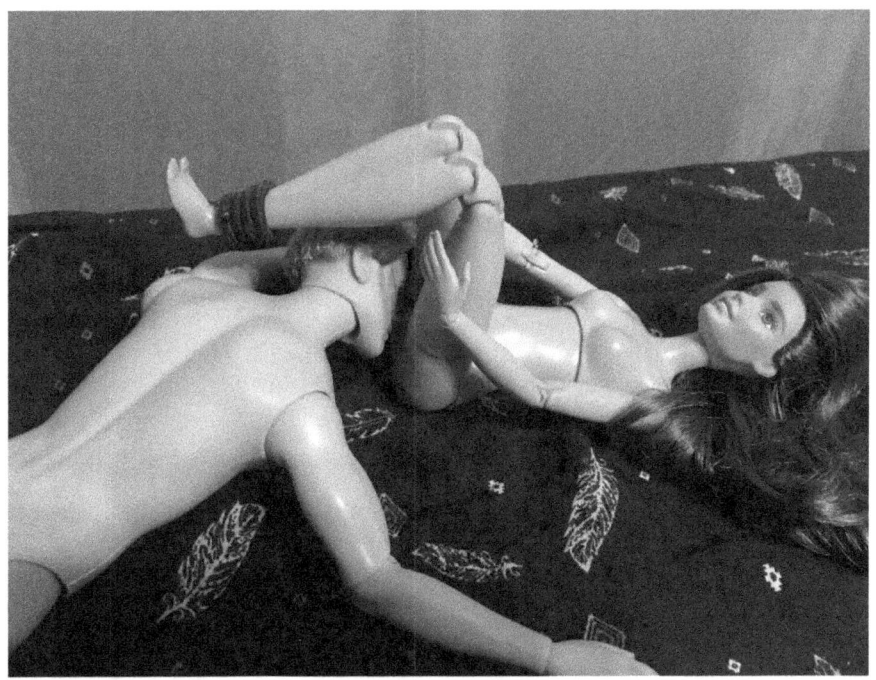

Picture 23 Cunnilingus Spread Eagle

Captain Jack

Captain Jack is a great move for those less experienced in dominance. In this pose, the woman is the dominatrix and the man takes the position of the dominated. The position itself is dominating but if both of you are more comfortable you can add domination role play to enhance the situation.

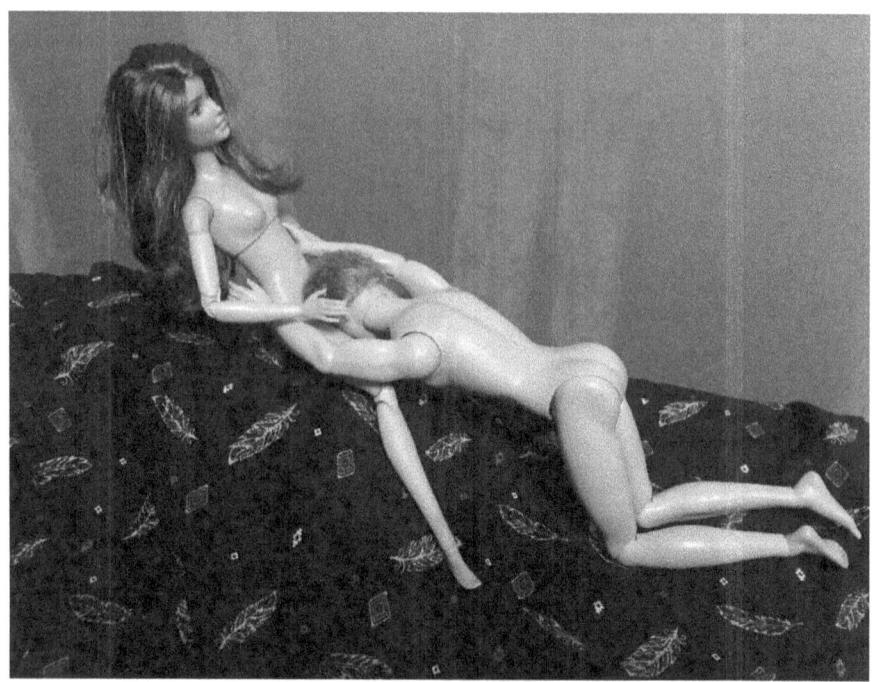

Picture 24 Cunnilingus Captain Jack

When you get to the pose, your woman will stand next to something that she can put her leg up on. It would also be good if there is something she can hold onto for balance. She will tell you to get on your knees in front of her. She may have to angle her pelvis forward so that you can access her vagina more easily. This pose is great for her to control the pressure and speed at which you eat her out. She can also grab your hair for added effect.

The Bridge

The Bridge is a sexy variation on the yoga pose. Have your woman start by lying on her back with her feet near her buttocks. Then she will press her hips up so that her pelvis is in the air. Help her spread her legs so that you can place yourself between them. Her vagina should be closer to your mouth and the position should make it so that it is more open. This pose can be very tiring so you might not be able to go down on her for that long. You can also help her by placing your hands on her lower back or buttocks and letting her rest on them. Because this is a strenuous pose she will probably not orgasm but that doesn't mean you can't have fun with it. She's more exposed and vulnerable so try to focus on her clit. This will create contrasting sensations. She will try to keep her legs strong but the feeling on her clit will make her weak.

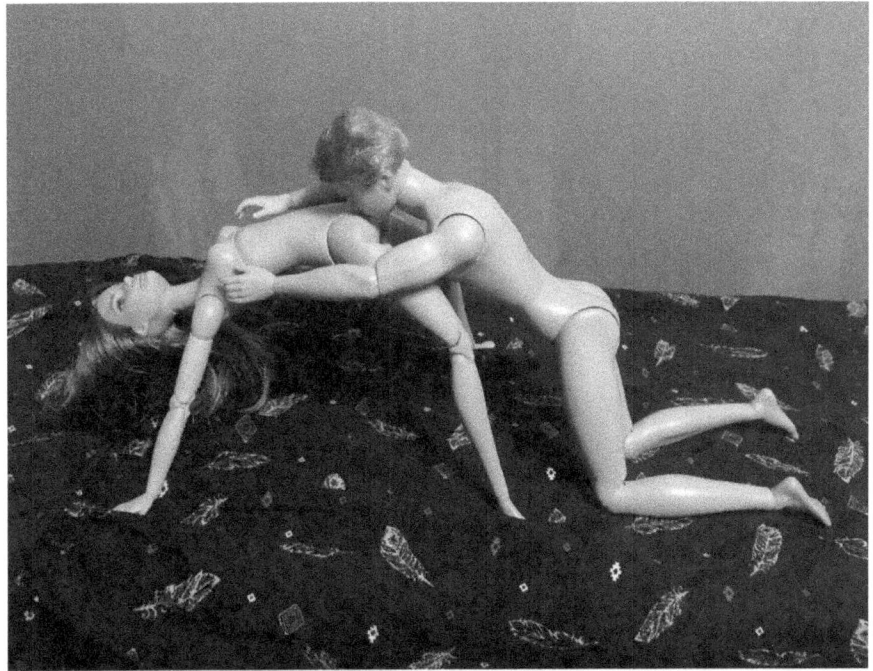

Picture 25 Cunnilingus The Bridge

Tip: You can turn this into a game. Have her try to keep her pelvis up as long as she can but at the same time use your mouth to make her collapse with pleasure.

The Backbend
Another sexual variation on a yoga pose. Have her attempt this pose, only if she's flexible and strong enough. Start by facing each other and then have her go into a backbend. When she's comfortable, spread her legs wide enough that you can position yourself between them. Again, you can help her by supporting her lower back and/or buttocks

with your hands. When you go down on her be more gentle. This position is not for teasing or for focusing on certain areas. Lick and suck her vagina as a whole. Make long, broad movements with you tongue and try to stimulate her vagina as a whole. You don't want to get her too riled up because this pose is very strenuous on her body.

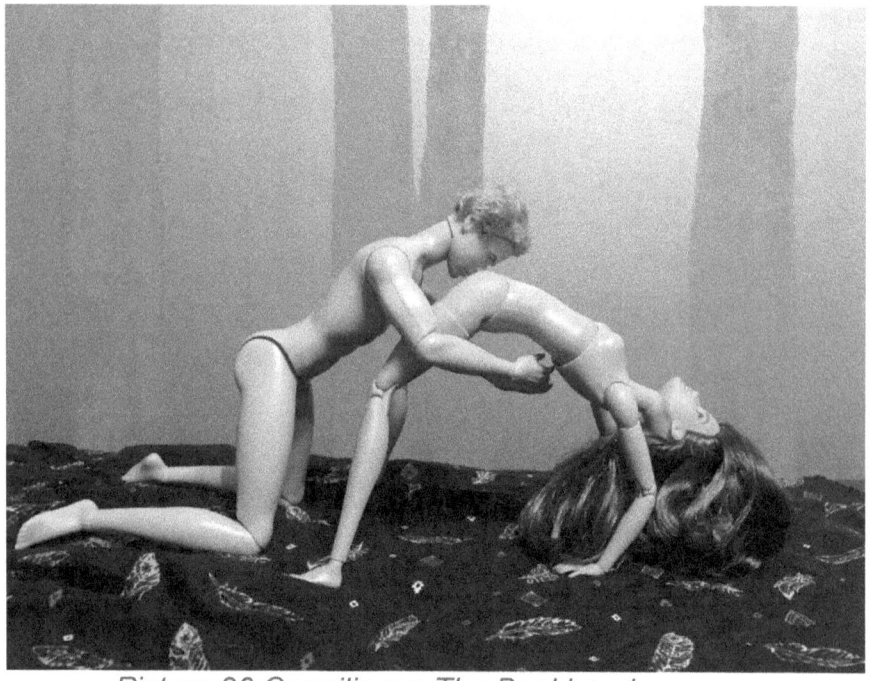

Picture 26 Cunnilingus The Backbend

The Ultimate Shocker

The Shocker is more of a move than a position but it's still great for stimulation. She can be in any position she likes but make sure she's comfortable. To do this move take your dominant hand and fold your 4th finger down (ring finger). Either lick your pinky finger or put lube on it because the anus doesn't produce any natural lubrication. Start by massaging her anus and loosening it up. Then slowly push your pinky into it while you insert your middle and index finger into her vaginal opening. For an added bonus you can take your thumb and rub it against her clit. In slow, fluid movements, begin inserting your fingers in and out of her vagina and anus. You can increase speed when she gets more comfortable and use to the sensations. While this is happening, lower your mouth onto her vagina and begin eating her out.

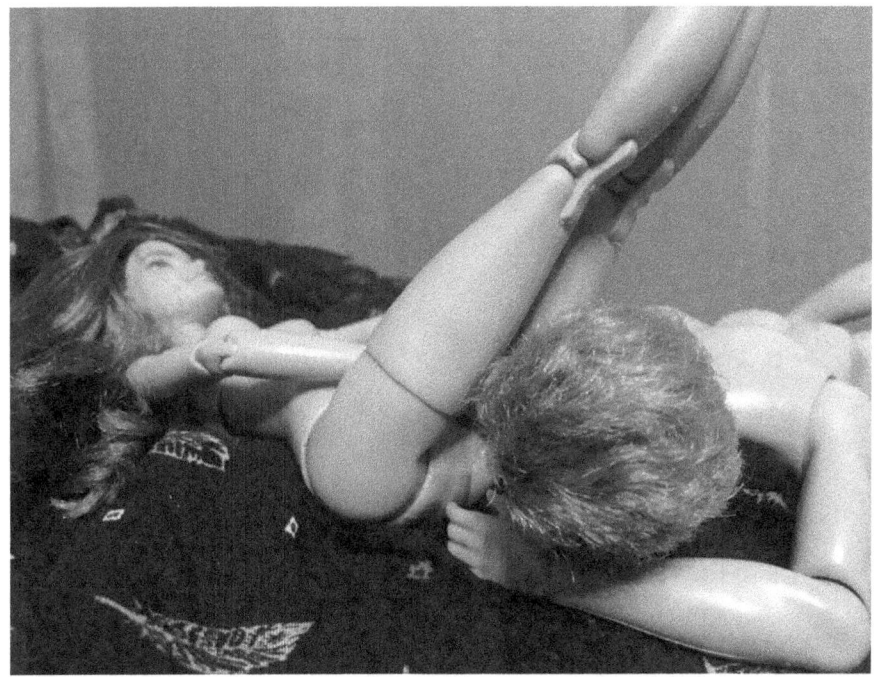

Picture 27 Cunnilingus The Ultimate Shocker

The Waterfall

This pose requires both of you to be in a shower. The warmth of the water and steam should help loosen her up so that she can feel the sensations on her vagina more intensely. Start by having her lean up against the wall, like in The Window Washer, but make sure the water is still hitting her back. Then proceed to go down on her. Angle your face so that you can breathe and water isn't entering your nasal passages. Try sliding your hands all over her body. The water should make her extra slippery. Make sure not to use soap before you attempt this position. It could slide down into her vagina and enter your mouth, which would be very unpleasant. Use this pose to really loosen her up. Instead of using your mouth intensely, try moving your tongue in a massaging fashion. The overall experience should be stimulating but at the same time, relaxing.

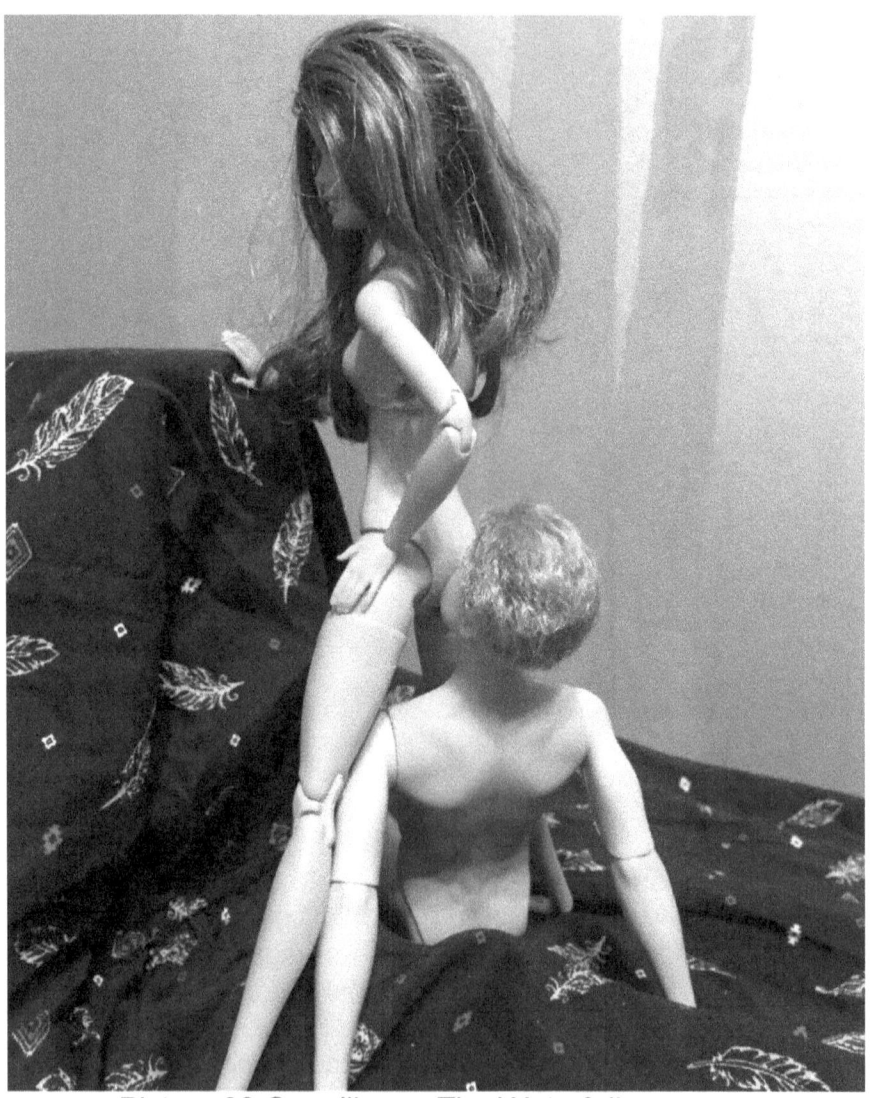

Picture 28 Cunnilingus The Waterfall

The Controller

This pose is very rough and dominating, so only attempt it if both of you are ready and experienced.

Communication is a big part of this move and it might be good to have a safe word. You will be taking the position of dominator and your woman will be the dominated. For this move you can put her in any position but the key idea is to be rough with her. While you're going down on her slap her breasts and/or butt. You can also try choking her, but make sure she's ok with it first. When you go down on her make it rough. Try biting her clit and the lips of her vagina. Use your fingers inside her vaginal opening and make sure to apply hard pressure on her clit with your tongue.

Tip: Have fun with it. Although this pose is all about dominance that doesn't mean you can't play around with it. Just make sure not to go past her limits. Have a conversation about this before you attempt this move.

The Balancing Act
This is a very advanced pose so only attempt it if you're strong and have good balance. You can also use a wall for assistance.

Begin on your knees. Have your woman get on your shoulders and then position herself so that your face is in her crotch. This is where the wall comes in handy. If you need help, have her lean her back against a wall, for balance, while you move into a standing position. It might be easier to do this if you support her with your hands on her buttocks. When you are both comfortable have her position herself so that her vagina is near your mouth. She may have to spread her vaginal lips for you to have better access. She can also grab onto the back of your head for support. This position is very tricky and doesn't allow for a lot of movement. Remember to only attempt this move if you're experienced with more advanced sexual positions.

These poses are only beginning suggestions for you to spice up your sex life. Use them to open each other up to new experiences but remember that you can add any variations you wish. Cunnilingus is meant to loosen your woman up for sex, so whatever you choose to do, make sure she's comfortable with it. And remember, take your time. Oral sex is a long journey, not a race.

Chapter 3: Fundamentals of BDSM Games

BDSM is a wonderful way for you and your partner to expand your sexual experiences. Many people have daunting thoughts when it comes to BDSM but when done correctly it can be very rewarding. One of the most important components is communication. You must be able to be open with your partner and communicate what you like and don't like. BDSM pushes your body to its sexual limits which is stimulating but can also be dangerous. Only attempt BDSM if both of you are open and ready.

BDSM consists of many different forms. They can range from relatively tame to more extreme forms. In this chapter, we will go over some different forms of BDSM and explain how to utilize them to gain the most sexual pleasure.

Shibari

This ancient Japanese technique of rope bondage originated around the 1400's with the name Hojo-jutsu. It started as a way for the Samurai to tie up and torture their prisoners while still showing them honor. Eventually, it evolved into an erotic form of bondage called Kinbaku or Shibari.

The idea of Shibari is to create patterns in the rope that work in contrast with the body's natural curves. The ropes and knots are arranged in such a way to emphasize sensuality, vulnerability and strength. By placing the knots in certain areas, the body's pressure points can be stimulated (very much like acupuncture). Shibari gives both people participating, a rush of endorphins and adrenaline. Many describe the experience to be extremely stimulating and even euphoric. There are even several exhibitions that relate to Shibari being considered an art form.

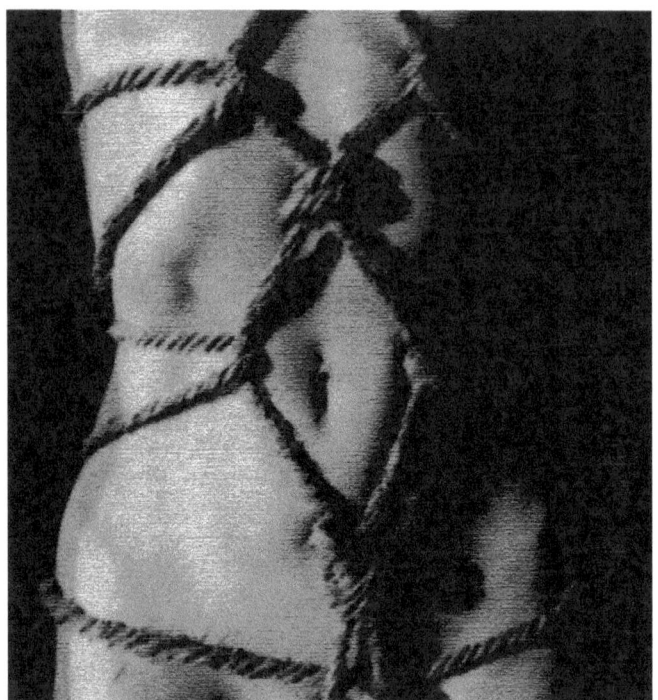
Picture 29 BDSM Shibari

This form of BDSM does not relate to those porn videos where you see someone tied to a chair. Shibari is a respected practice that isn't simply used for restricting movement. If you wish to experiment with Shibari make sure you really read up on it so you can be sure that you're doing it right. Many practitioners of Shibari say that it's not *what* you do but *how* you do it. There are many different ways to tie your partner so we've listed a few of the more common ways.

Equipment
- Natural fiber rope (hemp, nylon, or jute)
- Safety scissors (preferably EMT shears that can cut through rope quickly)
- Lotion

- The "Single Column" Tie: This tie goes around one thing (a wrist, ankle, bedpost, etc.)
- The "Double Column" Tie: This goes around two things (two wrists, two thighs)
- Chest Harness: Decorative tie that goes around the breasts (good for restriction and anchoring point)
- Leg Tie: Tie that restricts legs (forces person to kneel or keep their legs bent)
- Armbinder: Ties the arms and wrists behind the back (restrains movement in the whole arm and emphasizes the breasts)
- Cross Legged Ties: Ties the legs into a crossed position (gives support while restricting mobility)

There are many different tying techniques used in Shibari, these are just the basic few. If you're interested in this type of BDSM make sure you do your research thoroughly and find a partner who is willing to practice with you. Once you learn the basics of Shibari, you can move onto more advanced positions such as suspension. Remember to always be alert to your partners signs of discomfort and pain but also remember to have fun with it. Shibari is a beautiful art that can create intense sensations for both partners.

BDSM Sex Toys and Accessories

BDSM is most commonly known for its use of sex toys and accessories. Both men and women can enjoy the pleasure from these toys. Below we've listed some of the basic toys and accessories that can help spice up your sex life.

Blindfolds

Blindfolds are a great way to increase sexual stimulation without venturing deep into BDSM. By covering your partner's eyes, you increase their body sensitivity. The lightest touches are felt 10x stronger. You can use this with any variation of BDSM and it works great with all other toys.

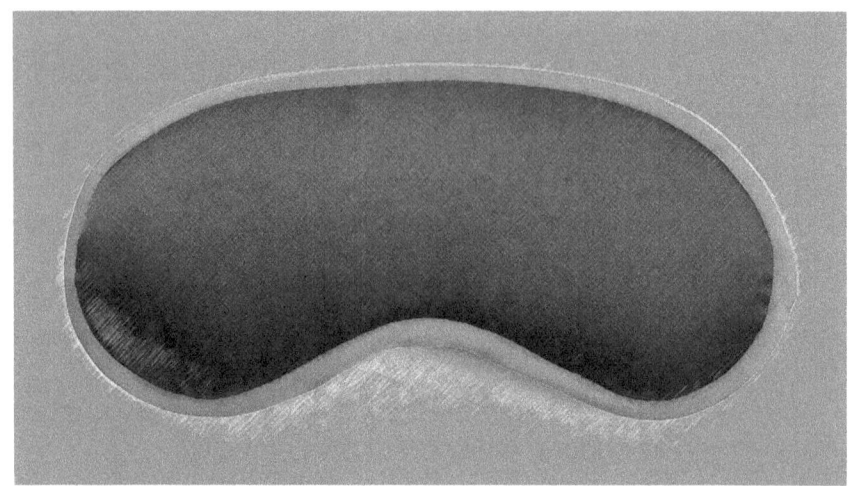

Picture 30 BDSM Sex Toys and Accessories Blindfolds

Gags

Gags are meant to go over the mouth and prevent your partner from making noise. They come in different variations. A plain gag simply goes over your partner's mouth and ties tightly behind their head. This keeps them from talking or making any loud noise. Ball gags have a ball in the center that goes inside your partner's mouth. The ball gag forces their mouth open but still restricts them from making much noise. Another variation of a gag has a hole in the center that allows you to slip your penis into their mouth but still restricts the amount of sound they can produce. Whichever gag you choose to use, make sure you and your partner are very familiar with each others limits. They won't be able to tell you to stop or utter the safe word so you must be able to read their body signals and know when they're at their limit.

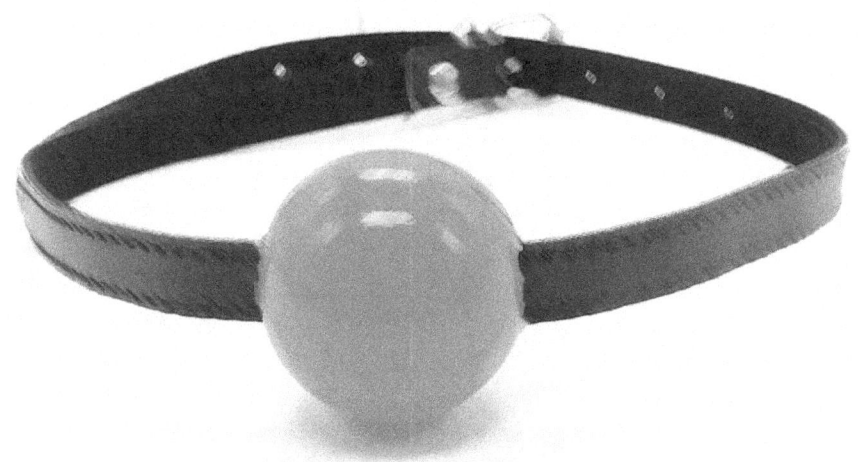

Picture 31 BDSM Sex Toys and Accessories Gags

Vibrators

Vibrators are silicone machines that emit strong pulses or vibrations used for stimulation. Men and women can benefit from vibrators. Women use vibrators to stimulate the inside of their vagina or the clitoris. One example is the popular Magic Wand. This vibrator has a multi-speed setting and is used for clitoral stimulation. Men can also use it as well. It offers intense stimulus to the outside of the penis and the area around the testicles.

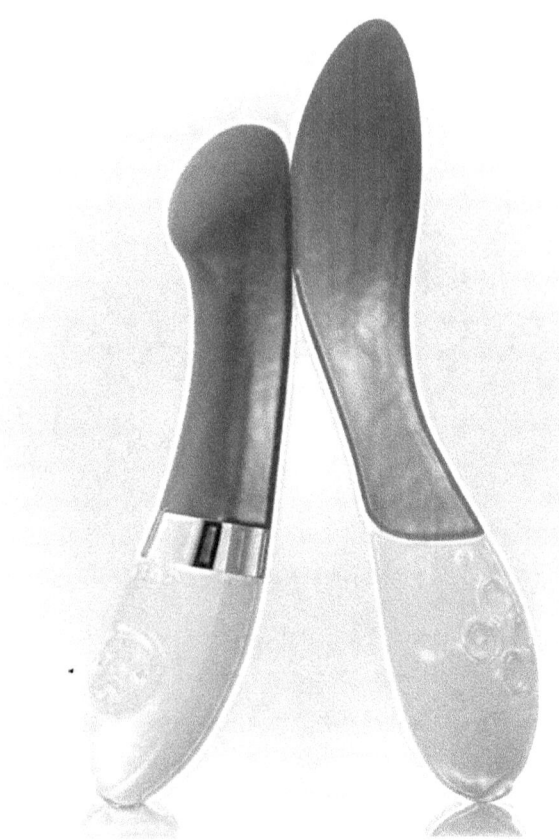

Picture 32 BDSM Sex Toys and Accessories Vibrators

Dildos

Dildos are silicone toys that resemble a penis. They're meant to mimic an actual penis in look and feel. They range in different colors to different sizes. Both men and women can experience pleasure from a dildo. A woman can use it to stimulate the inside or her vagina or even her anus. Men can derive anal stimulation from it. If you and your partner are open to using toys, the dildo can be a good beginning choice.

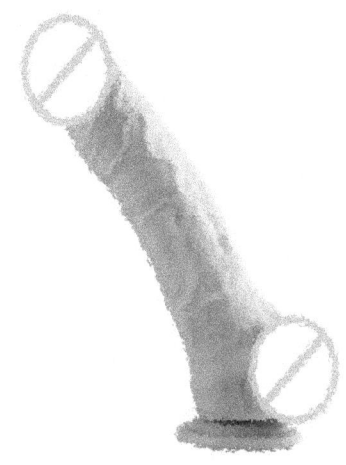

Picture 33 BDSM Sex Toys and Accessories Dildos

Cock Rings

The cock rings are specifically for the man's use. Cock rings are made of a semi-resistant material that slips over the man's penis and tightens around the base of his shaft. The restriction felt in the penis keeps him on the brink of orgasm and intensifies the sensation when he's released. Cock rings are a great form of basic bondage.

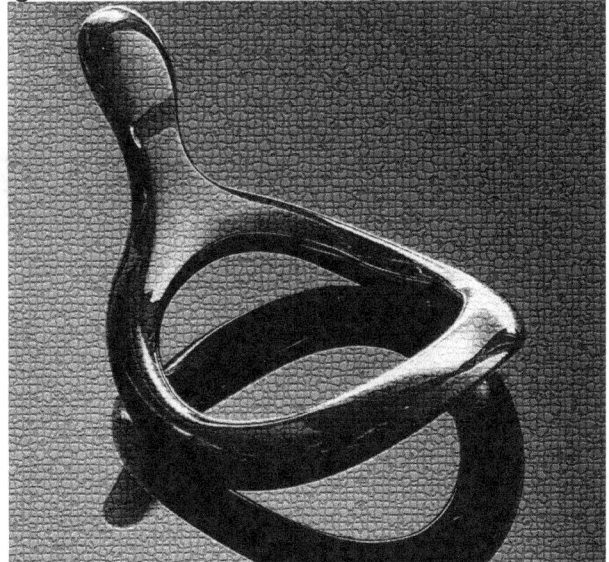

Picture 34 BDSM Sex Toys and Accessories Cock Rings

Butt Plugs

Butt plugs are amazing for sexual stimulation and they're also great for training to having anal intercourse. The anus is a very tight muscle that needs to be well stretched if you're ever planning on doing anal. Butt plugs come in different sizes which allows you to slowly increase the size of the object put in your butt. It also helps you get use to the feeling of having something go into your anus. There are many different styles of butt plug that work well for women and men.

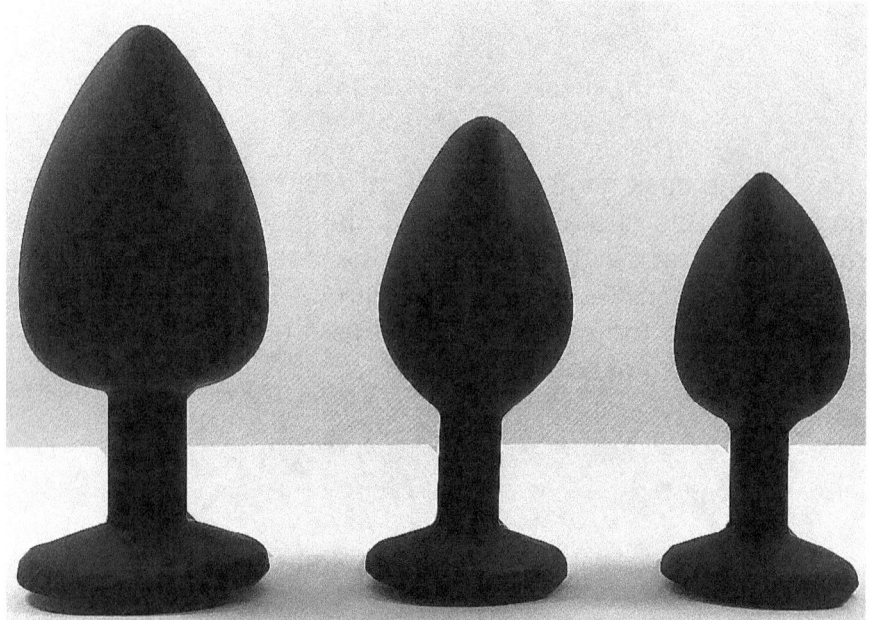

Picture 35 BDSM Sex Toys and Accessories Butt Plugs

Collars

Collars are a fun way of spicing things up in the bedroom. It can be worn by either the man or the woman or whoever the dominated person is. There are several styles of collar ranging from more chic and stylish to ultimate bondage. You'll find that many of the collars have a hoop at the end.

This is to attach a chain which can connect to the hands, the nipples or be left hanging and used in Master/Pet role play.

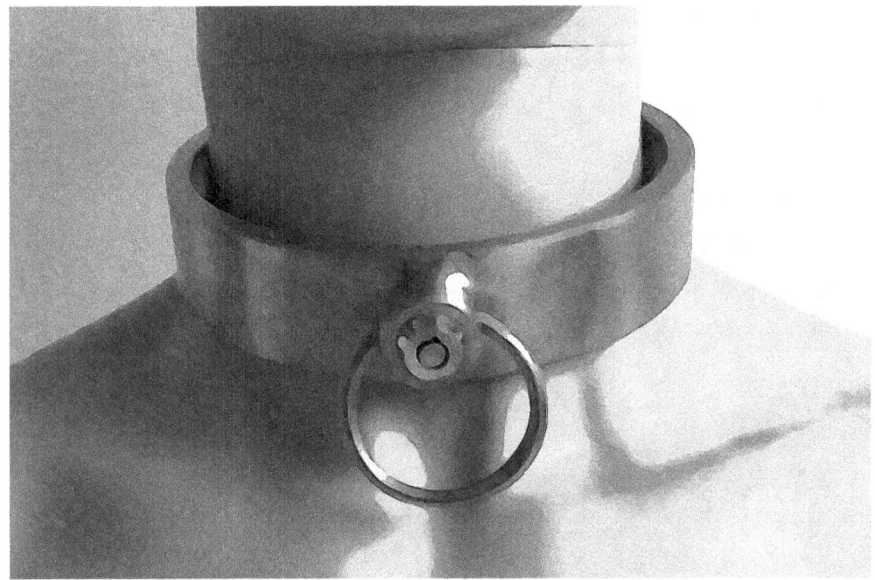

Picture 36 BDSM Sex Toys and Accessories Collars

Nipple Clamps

These are perfect for those that like a little more pain. Tweezer-like clamps are used to pinch the nipple in an arousing way. They are moderately tight so the pinching sensation can be intense for those not use to. Not only does it stimulate the nipples but when left on they can make the chest are more sensitive. There are clamps that dangle from the nipple, can be attached to a collar or even vibrate. If they are made of a soft enough material they can also be used on the clitoris.

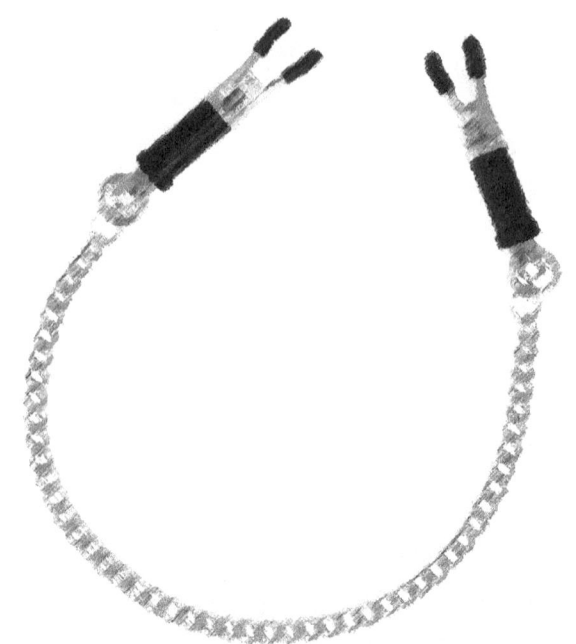

Picture 37 BDSM Sex Toys and Accessories Nipple Clamps

Whips/Paddles

This toy is the most associated with BDSM. Whips and paddles generally come in a soft leather material that stings but doesn't wound. A paddle is a harder material that doesn't give way. It's more ridge and therefore generally used for spanking. Whips are a little strong and produce a harder sting when hit. Floggers are a type of whip that contain several strips of leather at the end. It can be used as a feather or a whip. Generally, it's sting is a little lighter than an actual whip's. But all are used in the area of punishment.

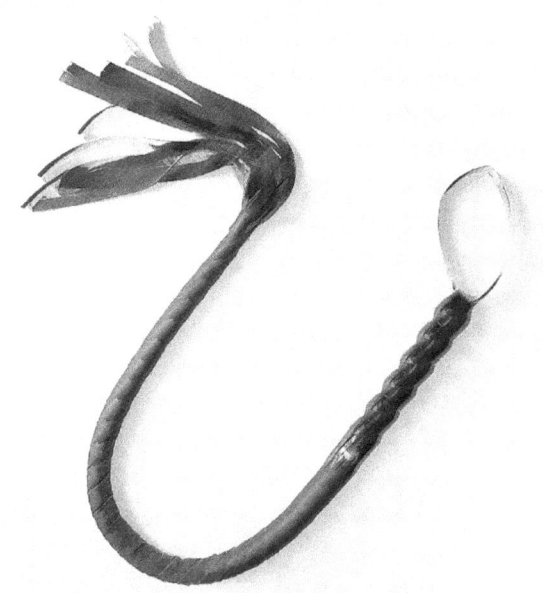

Picture 38 BDSM Sex Toys and Accessories Whips

Yokes/Ankle Spreaders

These accessories are designed to keep your limbs apart. Yokes are used for the arms and ankle spreaders for the ankles. Yokes look like a long bar that has wrist restraints on either side. It's meant to restrict arm movement and push the chest foreword so the breasts are emphasized. Ankle spreaders have the same concept with a bar and ankle restraints on either side. It's meant to restrict leg movement and keeps the thighs apart.

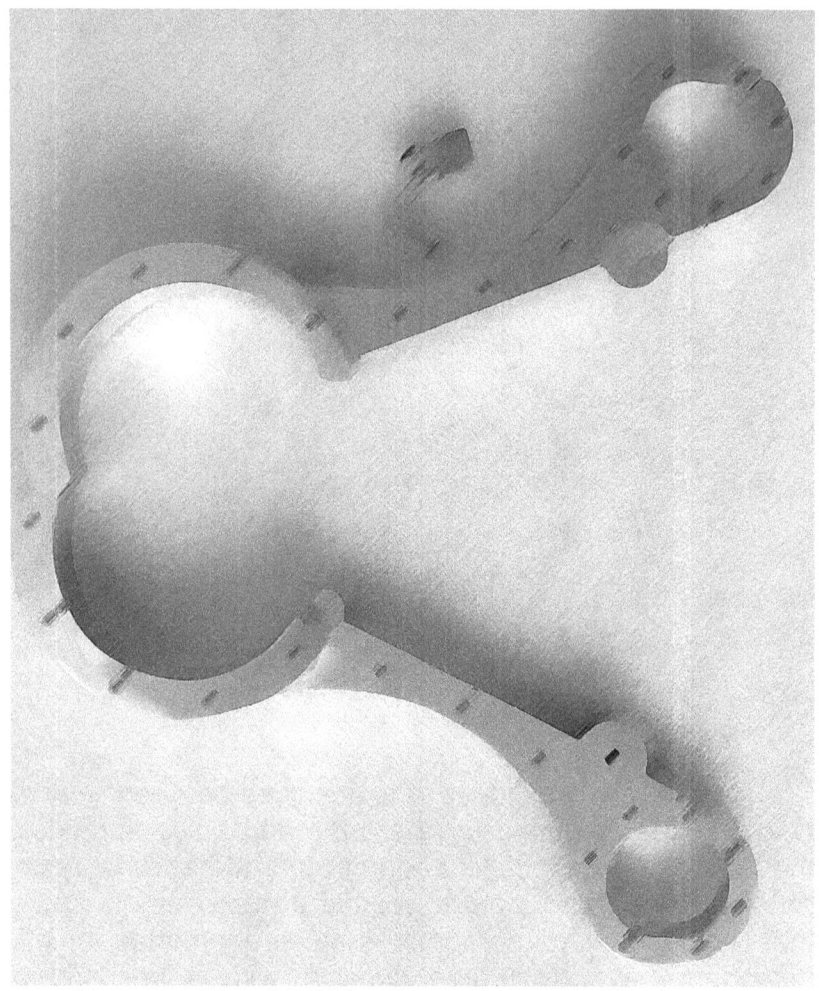

Picture 39 BDSM Sex Toys and Accessories Yokes/Ankle Spreaders

Striking Techniques

When it comes to using toys/accessories that involve striking, such as a whip, there are some things to take into consideration. This includes the type of impact, how to strike the blow, which parts of the body are the best to hit, how you can control the force of the impact. Striking can be dangerous and painful if not done correctly. But, it you learn the correct techniques, which we will go over in this section, it can be a very pleasurable experience for both you and your partner.

Different striking accessories have different impacts, even when used with the same amount of force. The most important advice is to start out by trying them out on yourself first and when you move to your partner start out gently (their pain threshold is probably not the same as yours). Here are some of the most common striking accessories and the types of sensations they produce.

- **Paddle:** The paddle is used for spanking (if you don't have a paddle you can also use your hand). You can use spanking anytime during your sexual experience to enhance sensations and even help your partner to orgasm. Spanking can be done lightly, as a playful move, or harder, as a type of punishment. Places that you can spank include: the face, the breasts/chest, the buttocks and the legs. If you choose to use a paddle make sure you reserve this only for the fleshier parts of the body, such as the buttocks. The paddle produces a harder more intense slap than the hand and is great to use during punishment.
- **Flogger:** The flogger is a type of whip that has many tails at the end. It produces a thudding type of pain that is less intense than a whip. It can be used as a tickler when trailed across your partner's body or a as whip when used with force. The flogger is best used on the fleshy parts of the body like the thighs or buttocks.
- **Whip:** A whip is like a flogger but with only one tail at the end. This makes the striking sensation more intense and almost like a sting. Whips can be hard to control and should only be used if you're really experienced. For the subordinate, the whip produces a very intense pain, so only enter into this area if you're comfortable with being struck and want a stronger sensation. Only use the whip on fleshy areas like the buttocks or thighs. (A whip can cause serious damage to the body if not used correctly.)

- **Caning:** A cane is similar to a whip but is made of a strong, flexible wood. It has a sharp and intense pain that will probably end up leaving a bruise or a welt. There are many different types of canes so it's up to you what type of material you use. Generally, they're made of natural fibers, like bamboo and synthetic fibers, like plastic. Canes must be cared for because they can splinter and cause serious harm to the subordinate.

How to Strike
When you're ready to use your whip on your partner, follow these steps to ensure their safety and pleasure.

- Tie them up so that they are perfectly still when you strike them. If they have room to move around it can cause the whip to hit somewhere it shouldn't or it can hit the body in the wrong way and end causing more pain than pleasure.
- Communicate. If your partner is going to strike you make sure you pay attention to what they're telling you to do. In turn, if you're going to strike your partner make sure they completely ready before you begin.
- As the person being hit, you need to mentally prepare yourself for what's going to happen. It's going to be painful the first couple of times. Eventually the adrenaline rush will kick in and then it will start becoming more pleasurable.
- If you are using a paddle, have them lay across your legs with their buttocks over your hips. Have them pick a number, which will be the number of spanks they receive. Bring down the paddle is a swift strong motion so that it smacks completely across their butt. Alternate between this and rubbing their butt with your hand. Rubbing it will help give them relief and cool down the stinging sensation. Make sure to take your time with this and enjoy it as much as they are.
- If you are using a flogger, begin by trailing it across their body. This helps acquaint them with the object. Then start swinging it in the form of a figure eight. Start out by gently rotating your arm in this pattern. When they're more

accustomed to it, tell them you're going to strike harder, and then bring your arm down harder as you continue making the figure eight. When you've got it down, start creating a rhythm. This can help move your partner from a painful sensation to a more hypnotic one. You'll want to make sure that the tips land on the body first so the tail doesn't end up wrapping around the body.

- If you are using a whip, there are many different ways to strike your partner. The most basic is the overhand. When whipping, you need to have a strong stance. This is so the whip does fly all over the place when you actually strike. Make sure your forearm and elbow move in a straight line and your hand ends up pointing to where the whip will land. Practice this a few times without your whip. When you think you've got it, hold the whip in your hand with a moderate grip. Pull your arm behind your head and try to extend it with the whip in one fluid movement. Practice this many times on an inanimate surface and only when you've managed to strike the same spot multiple times, can you try it on your partner.

- If you are using a cane, place it a few inches away from your partner's skin and flick it onto the desired area. Make sure to use the lower end but not the tip. The tip is sharp and can end up cutting through the skin. When your partner is comfortable with the sensations, move your hand further away and increase your swinging motion. It's important that you keep your hits parallel because crossing them can cause serious injury. Try alternating between a stinging and thudding sensation. This has to do more with the type of cane than the technique. A lighter cane causes a sting while a heavier cane causes a thud. Again, only use the cane on the fleshier parts of the body, like the bottom of the thighs.

- When you're finished, untie your partner and help them get up. Their skin is going to be very sensitive for the next couple of days so make sure you touch them very gently. It can also help if you rub lotion on the sore areas at least twice a day. Don't strike them again until their skin has completely healed.

The whip can be used to excite all parts of the body but certain parts of the body require different striking forces. In general, a whip can be used as a tickler on every body part. You simply take the whip and gently trail it over your partner's body so that they barely feel it. You can use this in the beginning to get them use to the feel of the whip and to arouse their sensitivities. The most sensitive parts of the body are the buttocks, the inner thighs, the stomach and the breasts/nipples. You can also very gently flick the whip, so that it lightly taps against these areas or any other area on their body.

When you've worked up to a full on strike, this is reserved only for the thicker parts of the body. This means you only want to strike your partner on the thighs, the buttocks and the breasts. This goes for both men and women. Again, this is also up to personal preference. Your partner might not like being struck on the breasts or the legs. Make sure you let your partner know where you're going to whip them and start with gentle force. If they are comfortable with the positioning, then slowly start increasing force. Each body part will require a different level of force. For instance, you're not going to strike the breasts as hard as you might strike the buttocks. You can also strike the genitals but make sure not to use too much force. A light smack will suffice to arouse your partner.

Warning: Be careful and avoid striking these areas: the lower back, kidneys, tailbone, hips, spine, neck, face and ears. Hitting these parts of the body can cause serious if not fatal damage. Also, make sure to set limits with your partner so you don't strike them in a place they don't enjoy. Vary your hitting techniques and also where you hit so the skin doesn't become tough and desensitized.

Controlling the Force

Controlling the force of your strikes is really something that comes along with practice. The more you strike your partner and figure out what they enjoy and what their limit is, the more it'll become second nature. The real key to enjoying striking techniques is to start slowly. You and your partner are both new to this so you'll need to figure out what it is each of you enjoy. Start with softer accessories such as your hand and work your way up to the more advanced things, like caning. Remember that each toy has its own sensations. So, when you decided to try out a new accessory, start from the beginning. Strike your partner very gently and work your way up from there. BDSM is all about exploration and the sexual satisfaction you can derive from pushing your body to its limits.

Sex Machines

If you're really looking to change things up in the bedroom, you may want to look into buying a sex machines. These are mechanical constructions that work in such a way that they mimic sex. There are also some machines that can be used by you and your partner to enhance your sex lives. Listed below are some of the most pleasurable machines you can buy and how you can use them to your benefit. Try utilizing these machines along with other techniques you've learned throughout this book.

The Wand Cushion

If you're a big fan of the magic wand this is for you. This cushion has a hole that allows you to place your wand inside so you don't have to hold it. For many, a tired arm hinders orgasm. It also allows you to sit comfortably with your clitoris placed directly onto the wand for maximum pleasure. This can work as a masturbation tool or it can help free your hands to pleasure your partner as you are being pleasured. If you're using it for masturbation, run your hands all over your body and stimulate areas that might not get much attention such as your nipples or even your head. If you're using it with your partner you angle the cushion so that your clitoris is stimulated while he penetrates your vaginal opening or your anus.

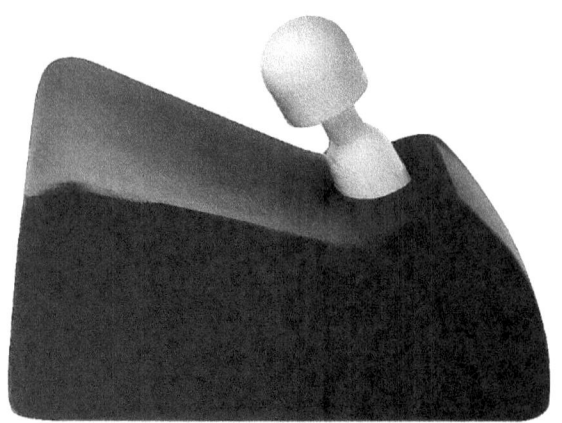

Picture 40 Sex Machines The Wand Cushion

Dildo Machine

The dildo machine comes in many variations but the concept is the same. A dildo is attached to an arm that thrusts at various speeds. Mainly, it's used for masturbation but it can also be used for intercourse. You can interchange the type of dildo for different sensations and you can also control the speed and power at which it thrusts. Generally, you have to be on all fours but some machines offer incline changes that allow for different positions. This is great if you're by yourself but still want to mimic the feeling of sex or if you want a more powerful thrust. But you can also use it with your partner for intercourse. You can perform cunnilingus or fellatio on whoever is using the machine.

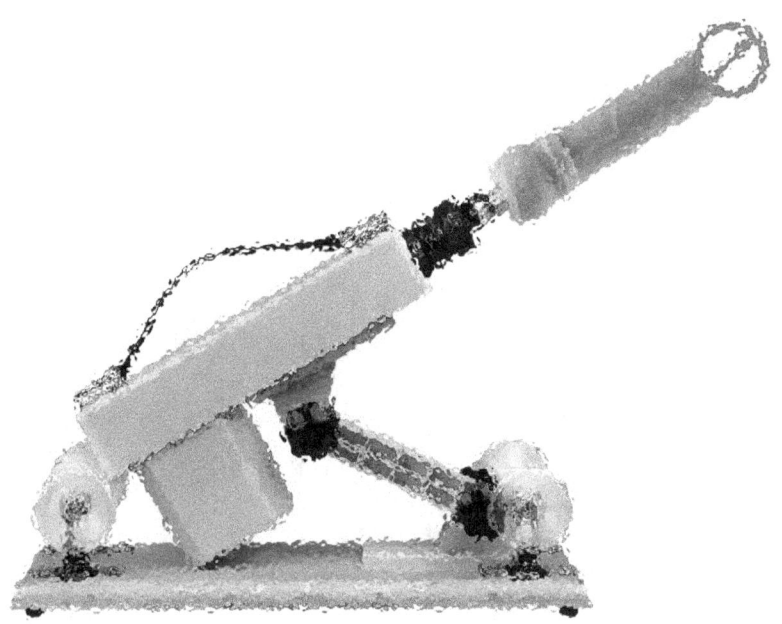

Picture 41 Sex Machines Dildo Machine

Rider

Riders are like dildo machines that you sit on. There are two soft pads that you straddle with a dildo in between. The seat is constructed so that as you move forewords and backwards the dildo thrusts in and out of your vagina. This is great because it allows you to control the speed and depth with your own movement. It also provides a more realistic felling of sex than the dildo machine. You can use it on your own for masturbation or even for intercourse. Have your partner sit in front of you and watch while you ride this machine to an orgasm. This also allows you to perform cunnilingus or fellatio as you're being pleasured.

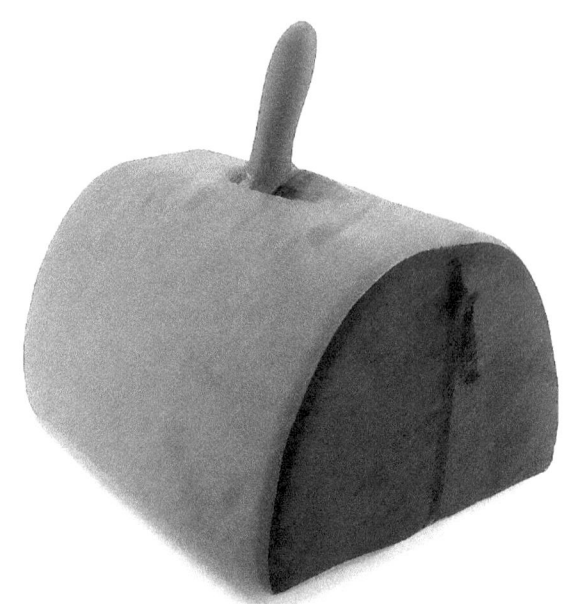

Picture 42 Sex Machines Rider

Sex Swing

A sex swing is a type of harness/hammock that suspends one person in the air. It allows for a bigger range of motion and deeper penetration. Typically, the woman sits in the swing while the man stands in front. You can use the swinging motion to thrust deeper and faster. It also allows the woman's legs to be spread further apart which allows the man's penis to go in deeper. You can also use the swing to perform fellatio and cunnilingus. It is even a great tool that allows those with disabilities a broader range of sexual activities. If you have a hard time standing or don't have the use of your legs, the swing is great for letting you experience the sensations created through different positions.

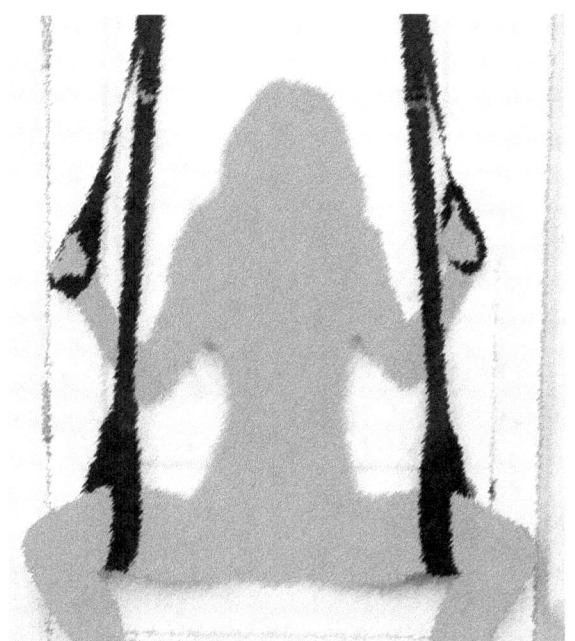

Picture 43 Sex Machines Sex Swing

Fuck Lounger

The fuck lounger is a great machine for intercourse. It allows both you and your partner to recline comfortably on an inflatable bed. It's great for getting into comfortable positions for sex that help increase range of motion and deeper penetration. But, it also comes equipped with a dildo stand that allows for double penetration. Have your man recline onto the lounger while you straddle him. Lower yourself onto his penis while simultaneously putting the dildo into your anus. Double the pleasure for double the fun.

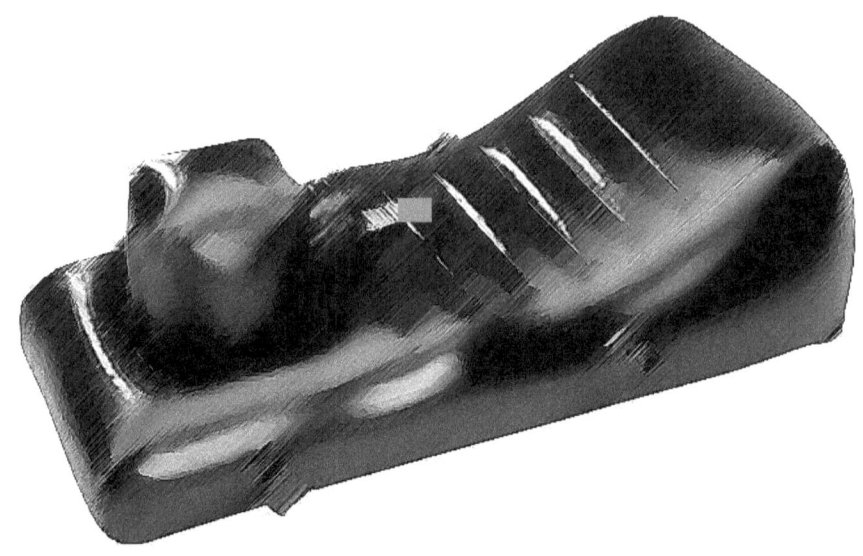

Picture 44 Sex Machines Fuck Lounger

Role Play

Role Playing is a great way to incorporate different forms of BDSM into your sex life. If you're not really for using toys or being tied up, role play allows you to spice up the bedroom through stimulating scenarios and dirty talk. If you're for it, It's also a great way to incorporate other aspects of BDSM, such as Shibari or even utilizing some accessories. Role play involves you and your partner pretending to be different people in a certain scenario. This can involve anything but it helps enhance the situation if you are in costume. We've listed the top 5 most common role playing scenarios to help you get an idea.

Teacher/Student

Teacher/student role play is one of the most well known sex scenarios. It involves one of you playing the teacher and the other the student. The teacher tells the student that they are failing the class and must do something to get their grades up. The student offers a sexual suggestion, such as oral, as a way to pass the class. Make sure you use a lot of dirty talk and flirting movements to enhance the situation. Use this scenario to incorporate some moves from the oral sex chapter, like The Boss or The Prayer. This role play is tamer and doesn't require the use of any toys. Feel free to incorporate them if you feel like it.

Tip: Use toys that fit into the scene for a more immersive experience. For example, a ruler is a great accessory to use for spanking.

Plumber/Housewife
The plumber/housewife is another role play that's suitable for beginners. There are many different variations of this scene that work just as well. (Repairman, delivery guy, postman, etc.) The idea is that a stranger comes to your house to do something and you need to repay them. Taking the plumber/housewife scenario: the plumber comes to the house to fix a leaky faucet and when he/she is finished the housewife or husband doesn't have any money to pay them. So, they must think of another way. This scene can be used to incorporate many of the different oral sex positions listed in Chapter 2. It is also a great way to have sex in other rooms of the house. Get out of the comfort zone of having sex in the bedroom.

Famous/Groupie
This is a really fun role play that you can get really creative with. One of you gets to play a famous person (actor, singer, DJ, etc.) and the other plays a groupie or super fan.
Whoever plays the star acts aloof and distant while the groupie tries everything they can to have sex with them. This is a great role play to practice flirting and foreplay. The star should try to resist the groupie for as long as they can. Really make them work for it.

Tip: If you're role playing the groupie try getting creative with your flirting. One thing that works really well is giving them a sexy dance. This role play is more about actions than dirty talk so utilize body movement as much as you can. If you're playing the star alternate between giving in and keeping away. Tease the groupie, make them sexually frustrated until you can't take it any longer. Then pounce and have some really great sex!

Master/Pet

In more advanced BDSM, master/pet role play is one of the most well known scenes. Generally, the man plays master and the woman pet, but you don't necessary have to do this. This role play is great for using toys and more advanced forms of foreplay. If you're more accomplished with Shibari, this role play goes great with the art of rope bondage. Only do this role play if you and your partner have a longer sexual history and you know each others sexual limits.

The master takes the dominating role and the pet the subordinate. You can choose to make the pet an actual animal (using toys with tails, ears, etc.) or you can simply be a subordinate. The master then commands the pet to do whatever he/she so desires. The adrenaline rush that you get from dominating and be dominated is what makes this role play so great. If you're the master, try using The Head Fuck when they perform fellatio or The Captain Jack for cunnilingus. This scene is great for using techniques learned for spanking, whipping, etc. But remember, although this role play is about domination it doesn't mean you should demean your partner. You must always have sexual respect for your pet.

Tip: If you're pet is really enjoying a certain stimulation, remove it before they orgasm. This role play is all about torture in the form of teasing. Bring them to the brink of orgasm but don't let them fall over.

Intruder/Victim

This role play is only for those that have practiced BDSM seriously. You must know your partner's sexual tastes completely. It's also important, for this role play, to have a safe word if you're really going to get into the scene.

One person plays the role of an intruder and the other plays the victim. The victim catches the intruder in his act of breaking in, robbing, etc. and threatens to call the police. The intruder then moves to "rape" the victim. This role play is very aggressive and can involve tying up, choking, toys (such as blindfolds) and anything else you wish to use. Gags especially, are a great accessory for this role play. This role play really lets you push each other to your sexual limits. Try using some striking techniques and really go for it (unless your partner says the safe word). The great thing about this role play is both of you can push each other to your sexual limits which ultimately leads to some really great rough sex.

Tip: A safe word allows you to try new things without having to stop and ask if it's ok. Do whatever you want to do and if they say the safe word then immediately stop. Use this to explore some of your deeper fantasies.

Part II: The Main Act

Chapter 4: The 10 Most Unusual Poses

Sometimes sex can get a little monotonous, making it a chore rather than a pleasurable experience. This usually happens to couples that stick to one routine and/or the same basic positions, such as missionary or doggy style. The key to having really great sex is mixing things up. Try something you've never done before, like BDSM. And if you're not into things like that, simply try a new position. Below we've listed the ten most unusual positions. They may be strange and even hard to get into but they're guaranteed to spice up your sex life and give you a great orgasm!

Tip: Make sure the woman is really lubed up to make getting into these poses a lot easier.

The Pile Driver
Start by having your woman either get into a headstand or a variation where she's on her neck and her legs are in the air. She can use a wall for balance and support if she needs to. Then, stand behind her so that her buttocks are facing your crotch. Open her legs as far as you want or as far as she is able and slowly insert your penis into her vagina. You may need to angle your penis down so that it can enter comfortably. Start out slowly with this position and adjust whatever you need to, to get comfortable. This position allows the penis to rub hard against the vaginal walls and go really deep, so as to hit the g-spot. It can be quiet strenuous on the woman so make sure you don't thrust too hard. It can also help if you put a pillow or something soft underneath her head or neck.

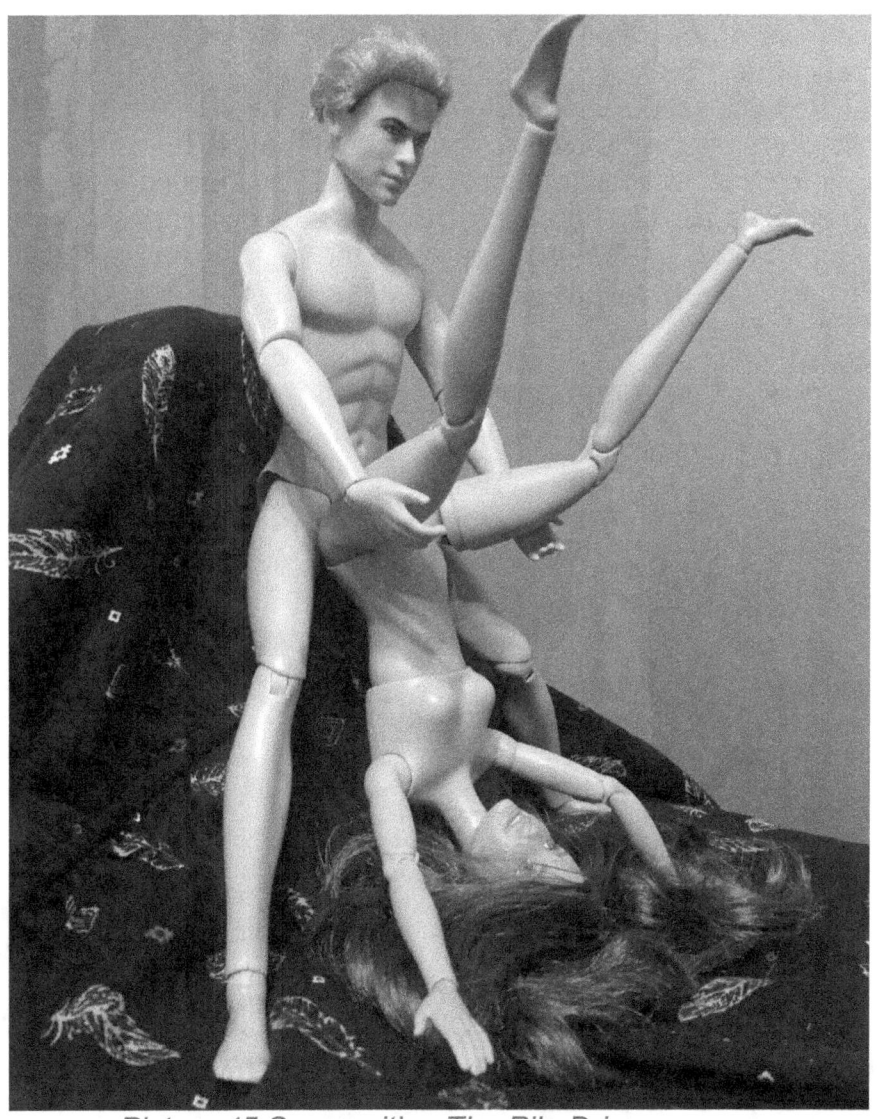

Picture 45 Sex position The Pile Driver

Neck Breaker

This pose is another variation of The Pile Driver and requires lots of flexibility in the woman. Start by having her go into the pile driver on her neck but instead of her legs going in the air, she should drop them behind her head so that her toes touch or come near to the ground. If she's flexible enough she can also drop her knees down beside her ears. Come up behind her, like you would in The Pile Driver, and squat down so that you can insert your penis into her vagina. This pose is also very strenuous on the man because he has to squat quite low to thrust so only attempt this if you have strong legs and good balance. By dropping her legs behind her head, the woman changes the angle at which the penis enters and hits. It makes the sensations very intense, which feels great for both partners!

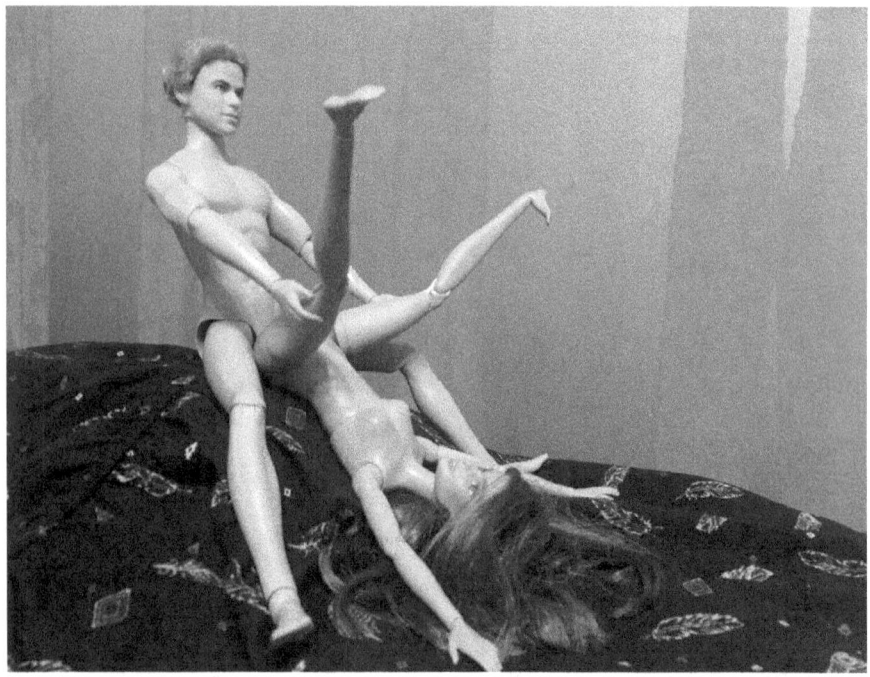

Picture 46 Sex position Neck Breaker

The Crab

The Crab is a really interesting pose and can be quite hard to get into. Start by having your man sit with his knees up and his hands close to or slightly behind his buttocks. Have him spread his knees and then maneuver yourself so that you can sit on top of him and insert his penis into your vagina. Place your hands close to or slightly behind your buttocks and have your feet planted on the floor. When you're both read, push up so that your body forms a flat surface, like a table. Then, have him try sliding his penis in and out. This pose can be strenuous for both of you so only attempt it if you have good balance and strong arms/legs. It can also put a lot of strain on the penis because it's being bent in an extreme angle. You can try this pose for a couple minutes but it probably won't lead to any orgasm.

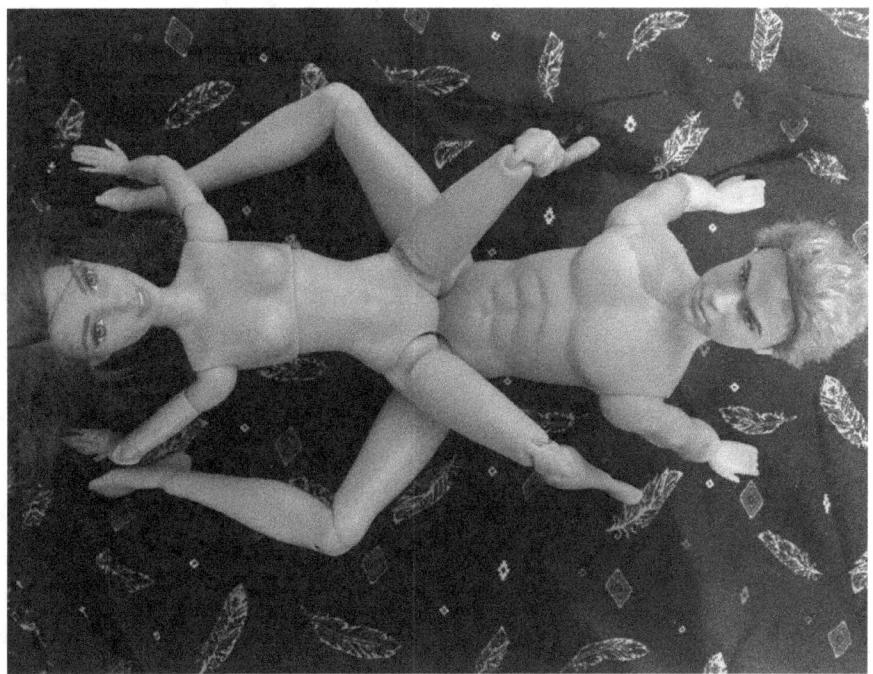

Picture 47 Sex position Crab

The Skydiver

The Skydiver is a fun move once you figure out how to position yourselves. Start by having your woman lie on her back. Turn yourself so that your face is near her feet and your belly is on the ground. Then, lie on top of her and angle your penis down so that you can insert into her vagina. You can also get into this pose by starting in missionary and rotating yourself with your penis already inside. Once you're in the correct position, lift yourself up slightly and begin thrusting in reverse. This pose feels great for the man because of the angle in which it's being bent and because of how it hits the vaginal wall. Your woman can also try angling her hips up to get a better angle at hitting the g-spot and to increase the pressure felt around the penis.

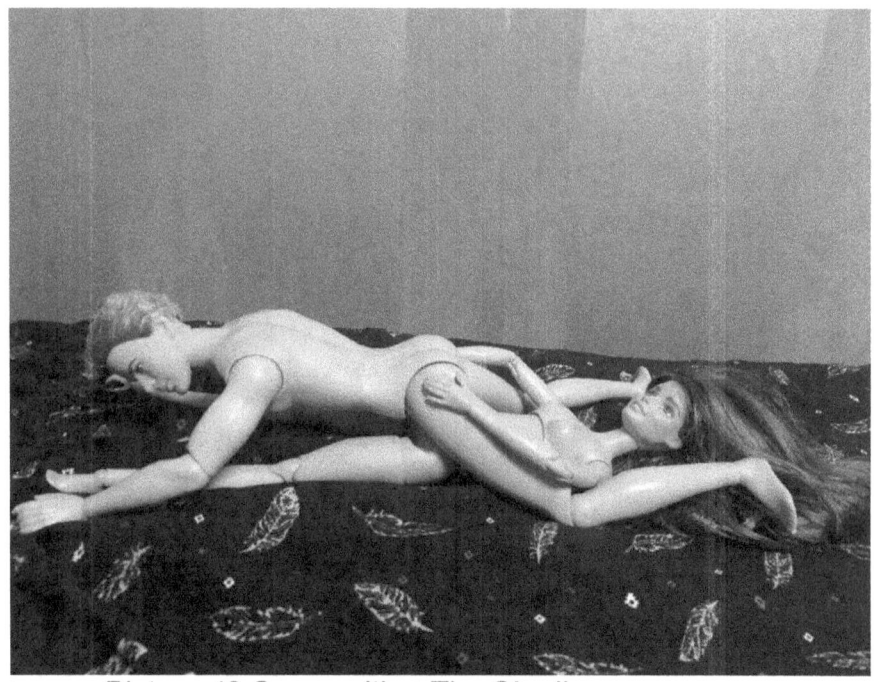
Picture 48 Sex position The Skydiver

Niagara Falls

This pose is very easy to get into and feels great for both partners. Have your man sit on the bed with his back facing the edge. Then, have him slowly bed backwards so that his head is touching the ground but this crotch and legs are still on the bed. When he's comfortable, come to the edge and lower yourself onto his penis so that your sitting on the edge of the bed and straddling him. This pose is great for the woman to control the speed and power of each thrust. Make sure to not thrust too hard or both of you might slip of the bed. It can be strenuous on your man's head and neck so place a pillow underneath for comfort. It can also help keep him from sliding around so much when you thrust. This pose also gives a great angle for the man. He can see practically see everything that's happening!

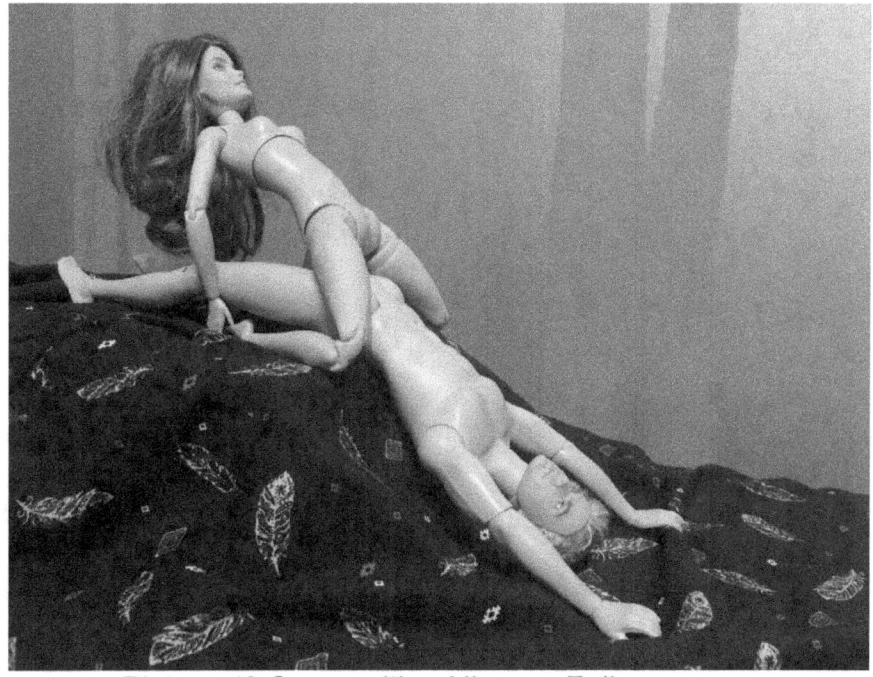

Picture 49 Sex position Niagara Falls

Chair Master

For the Chair Master you're going to need something that both of you can sit comfortably on. Start by having your man sit in a chair in a reclining position. Then facing him, sit on top and insert his penis into your vagina. When you are comfortable slowly lift one of your legs up and rest it against his shoulder. Then the other. You can either have them bent over his shoulders or if you're more flexible you can keep them straight in the air. Your man can begin thrusting by lifting you up slightly or you can rock your hips back and forth to rub his penis on the inside of your vagina. This move is great for getting really deep and for tightening the vagina wall around the penis. Make sure you warm up your legs with some stretches before you attempt this move or you could pull a muscle.

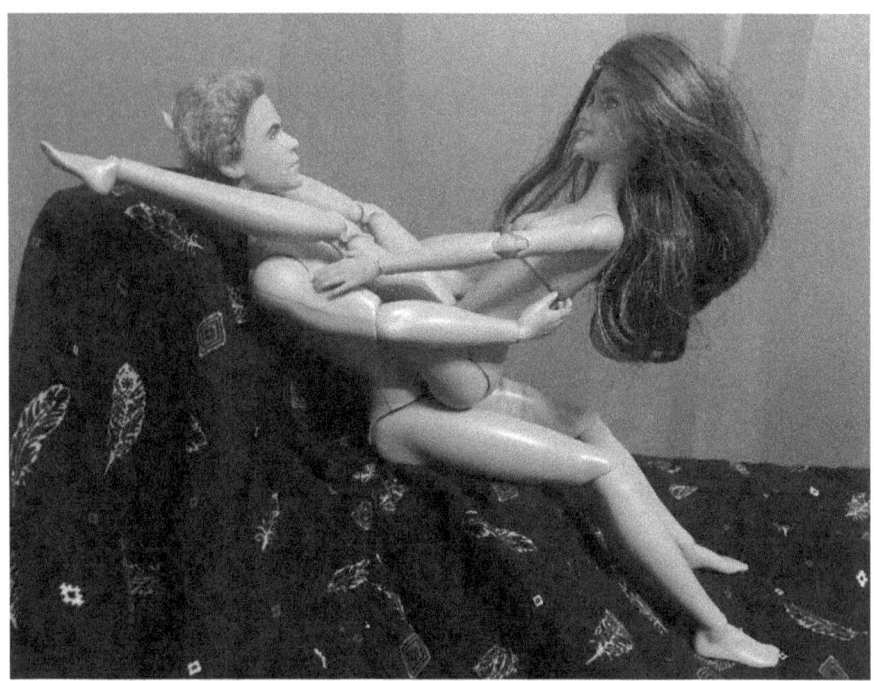

Picture 50 Sex positions Chair Master

The Eagle

The Eagle should only be attempted if you and your partner are very strong and have really good balance. Start by having your woman bend over a surface, like the bed. Stand behind her and insert your penis. Then, have her flex her whole body tightly, especially her core. Tell her to lift her legs off the ground and press them against your thighs while you put your hands on her hips. When you have a good, strong grip lift her up so that she's at a 45-degree angle. You can also have her place her hands on something to hold herself up and give you better stability to thrust. This move is very hard to do, so don't worry if you neither of you end up reaching orgasm.

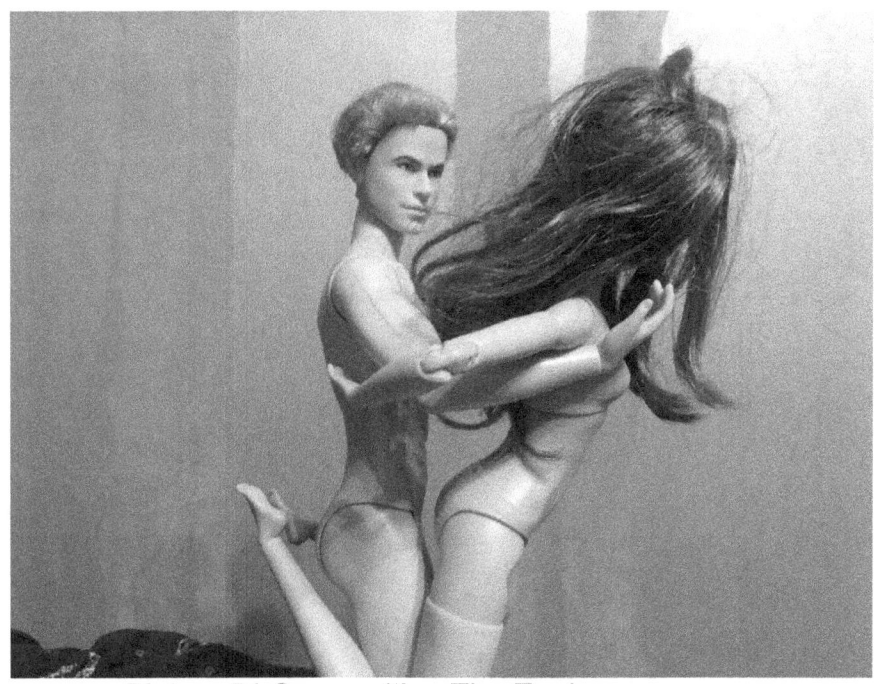

Picture 51 Sex position The Eagle

The Golden Gate

This move is like The Crab but only the man is in table top position. Your man can either go into table top or bridge pose (which requires a little more strength and flexibility). When he is in position, stand over his crotch so that you can lower yourself onto his penis. Make sure not to put your full weight on him or he could fall. This position is nice because you can either use your legs to thrust him in an out of your vagina. Or you can rock your hips back and forth to create a nice sensation from the friction between your two bodies.

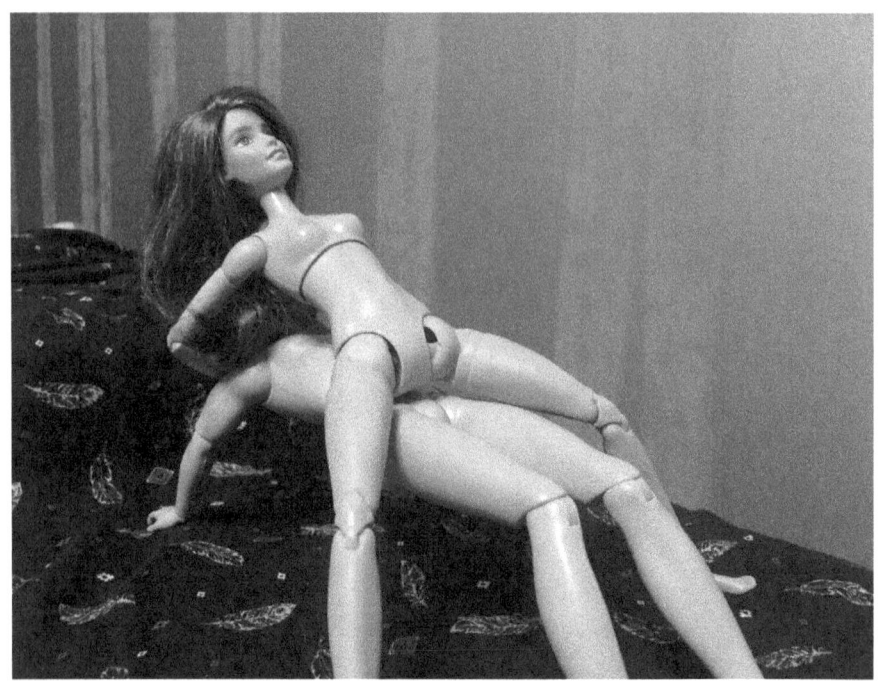

Picture 52 Sex position The Golden Gate

Tip: You can also reverse yourself so that your back is facing his face. This changes the angle of where his penis hits and is a great position to hit your g-spot.

The Ballerina

Like a ballerina, the woman must be extremely flexible for this position. Start by lying on your back. Have your woman sit on you and insert your penis into her vagina. When both of you are comfortable she can extend her legs to the side so that she is doing the splits, perpendicular to your body. You can either thrust your penis in and out or you can have her rock her hips back and forth. This pose can get very deep so give her time to adjust to the feeling. Also, make sure she stretches her legs and that you don't move to roughly or you could end up causing injury to her leg muscles. As with the previous pose, she can also reverse herself so that she is doing the splits with her buttocks pointing towards your face.

Not only does this move feel great but it offers a good view as well.

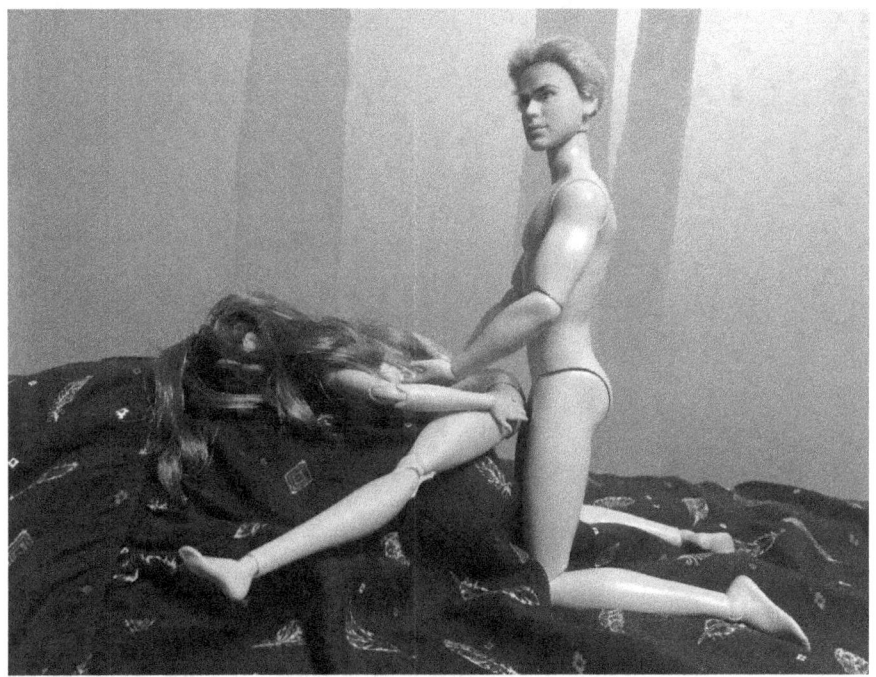

Picture 53 Sex position The Ballerina

The Geometrist

This position also involves the woman doing the splits. Have your woman lie on her right side. Then, with the right leg remaining on the bed have her spread her left leg as far into the air as possible. Position yourself so that your right knee is on the bed and your left is up (with your foot on the bed). Take her leg that's in the air and brace it against your body or with your hand. Lower yourself so that you can insert your penis into her vagina and begin thrusting. This is a very deep move so begin slowly and work your way up. You can also try stretching her leg further if she is comfortable. This widens the vaginal opening and allows for more range of motion. Just make sure you don't over extend her leg and strain her muscles.

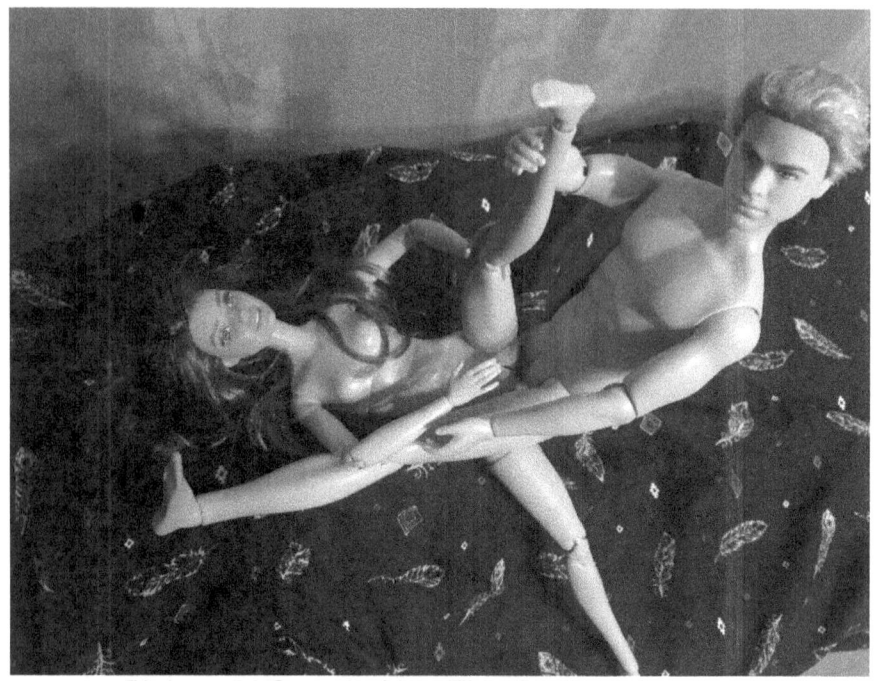
Picture 54 Sex position The Geometrist

Remember that these poses are not for everyone. Many of them are extremely hard to get into and require a lot of strength and balance. The point of these moves is to help you experiment and break out of old sexual routines. There are hundreds of different positions for you and your partner to experience. Try mixing several different moves during intercourse and you'll realize just how amazing the sexual journey can be!

Chapter 5: Squirt Technology

Getting your woman to squirt may seem like an impossible task, but it can actually be fairly easy. First of all, it's important to know that women have several different types of orgasms. There's the clitoral orgasm, the vaginal orgasm and the squirting orgasm. The clitoral orgasm is achieved by directly stimulating her clitoris with your finger or your mouth. The clitoris is highly sensitive so it's very easy for a woman to achieve this orgasm and there are many that have only ever experienced this type of orgasm. The vaginal orgasm is achieved by coming close to or hitting the g-spot. This orgasm is very intense and can be felt throughout their whole body but it's harder to make a woman get to this point and many have never experienced a vaginal orgasm. If you are able to make your woman orgasm in this way, then it's actually possible to give her multiple orgasms by stimulating the same spot. The squirting orgasm is when her g-spot is stimulated so much that she actually squirts out liquid from her vagina. This liquid is much like the cum that leaves a man's penis and it's not to be confused with pee.

Tip: To get your woman to squirt make sure she is comfortable with you and excited with the idea otherwise it will not happen. But also remember that not all women are squirters. While this method should help your woman achieve a squirting orgasm it's not guaranteed this will happen. So as always, just remember to have fun with it!

To start, make sure she is really lubed up along with your finger. It helps if you use a natural lubricant like coconut oil to make your finger really slippery. Then insert your finger and start with a technique called the clock. Flex your finger up so that it's pointing at "12 o'clock". Stay there and slowly move your finger up and down, like your massaging that one area. Then angle your finger so it's pointing to "1 o'clock", and so on and so forth. Keep doing this until you've gone all the way around and returned to "12 o'clock". This should help get her more relaxed and make her vagina more sensitive to your finger movements. It can also help if you give a simple vaginal orgasm first.

Next, you're going to try to locate the g-spot. It's located 1-2 inches inside the vagina at the top. It feels kind of like a sponge with some bumps and ridges. The more aroused she is the more pronounced it will become. (The clock technique and a vaginal orgasm should make it swell which will help you find it more easily). When you think you've found it start with a stroking technique. Move your finger back and forth in a slow short motion. Make sure you keep your finger firmly against the g-spot while you're doing this. Then, start building up speed and intensity. If she's really feeling the movement you can add another finger to enhance the pleasure.

If you've been stroking the g-spot correctly it should be pretty swollen by now. This is when you want to really increase the pressure and speed. Change your position so that your kneeling beside her with your back towards her face. Put the palm of you hand on her clitoris while your fingers remain inside. Then take your hand and move it up and down so that your fingers press on her g-spot while your palm stimulates her clitoris. Start building up speed and pressure until you're doing it as fast as you can and soon she should reach a squirting orgasm. It can be tiring for you arm and hand but if you really want her to squirt you'll need to keep up the same rhythm and pressure. If she doesn't squirt, it could just mean that she wasn't relaxed enough. For the woman, squirting feels a lot like peeing. This means that when they start to feel that sensation they often try to stop it. By placing a towel underneath, you can help to relieve some of the nervousness.

Some tips for the woman: Make sure you're completely relaxed when going into this. It can help if you pee before so you know there's nothing inside your bladder. Really get into what your man is doing. Not only does it help him feel like he's doing a good job but it helps you loosen up. Try not to keep any tension in your vagina as this could stop you from having any kind of orgasm. When it comes time to squirt you're going to feel pressure building up in your vagina around your g-spot. Because this is close to your bladder it's going to make you feel like you have to pee, but don't try to stop it. If you release the tension that's felt with the anxiety of possibly peeing, you can end up squirting!

Tip: If you manage to achieve a squirting orgasm through fingering then it's possible that you can achieve it through sexual intercourse. Continue with fingering until it feels more natural and then try to have your man use his penis to stimulate your g-spot in the same way and give you a squirting orgasm. Not only does this feel great for your man but it is really sexually liberating for the woman.

Chapter 6: Group Sex

For couples that are open to sleeping with other people, group sex can be a fun way to really change things up in the bedroom. Make sure you and your partner are really ok with the idea before inviting a stranger into your bed. There are lots of things to consider before committing to this idea. The person you invite is going to have sex with your man (or your woman). If you're not ok with this idea, then group sex isn't for you. So, if this doesn't bother you or your partner, then you're ready to "get it on"!

The first thing you really need to consider is who you're going to invite into your bed. Most commonly people start out with a threesome and work their way up to bigger groups. So, you need to decide if the person you choose is going to be someone you know or a stranger. Choosing someone you know is a lot safer but not always feasible so if you're going to choose a stranger, make sure you use protection.

Bringing this topic up isn't always so easier, especially if it's towards a friend. But it is possible. You could start by lightheartedly bringing up the subject of threesomes and ask them their opinion of it. If they seem to enjoy the idea, then you can start working your way towards inviting them to have a threesome with you and your partner. If it's a stranger, chances are you met them in a bar or club. This makes inviting them a lot easier especially if you've all had a couple of drinks.

Now, the person you've asked to join you and your partner has accepted and you're all in the bedroom! It can be a little awkward at first. Start by slowly taking turns kissing each other. This will help you all get acquainted with each others bodies and loosen you up. Sometimes it helps if one couple starts first while the other watches and then joins in when things start getting heated. Incidentally, group sex doesn't mean all people present have to participate.

Sometimes it can be fun just to have someone watching. There are also those that enjoy watching their partner have sex with others. It's really all up to what you and your partner are in the mood for.

If all three of you are participating in the act, make sure all of you have a role to play. Don't exclude anyone but also, don't be the person that just waits around for a turn. Threesomes are all about increased sensations. There's more hands and more mouths to offer pleasure. There are also many combinations: Three women; three men; two women and one man; and two men and one woman. We'll discuss these different combinations below and how they can offer different pleasures.

Three Women

Three women is a great threesome for lesbians, bisexuals or those who are just curious. This threesome generally has lots of toys involved to simulate penetration and make the experience more unique. The great thing about this threesome is each of you can perform cunnilingus on each other at the same time which is uniquely stimulating. Women can also be more pleasurable because they understand their own bodies. It's easier for them to take their time and explore each other before moving to penetration. When it comes to the actual act many of the toys used are listed in pervious chapters, such as a dildo or vibration. It can also include sex machines like The Rider. The Three Women threesome is really great if you are open to exploring your sexuality. It can also help you understand your own body more and help you find new ways to pleasure it.

Three Men

The Three Men threesome is exactly like Three Women but with men. So, if you are gay, bisexual or again, simply curious, this threesome is a great way to explore sex with men. A threesome with men can be very stimulating because of the fact that you can perform fellatio to one of your partners while they are being penetrated. Many men never experience the feeling of being sucked while penetrated and we've heard its an amazing experience. Toys can be involved in this threesome, like the cock ring, and even sex machines, such as the sex swing. Although, if you are new to this the simple act of intercourse should be enough to pleasure you. It's also good if all you experience being the bottom and the top, but this doesn't necessarily have to happen. In fact, many times there is a designated top and bottom while the other can go either way. Again, if you're new to this stick to what you feel comfortable with but try to make your way to experiencing both aspects of intercourse.

Two Women, One Man

This is one of the most common forms of a threesome and it's also a common fantasy for men. It can also be quite enjoyable for a woman. One of the benefits of this threesome is the man can step back and gain pleasure from watching his partner and another woman engage in intercourse. He can also have the opportunity of switching partners when he starts penetration. This is also a good position for focusing on one partner at a time. For instance, both women can perform fellatio at the same time on the man. Or the man and woman can focus on pleasuring the other woman. For example, while the man is penetrating one woman, the other can perform cunnilingus. This is also great to incorporate different positions, such as Dinner for Two. There's more diversity in this threesome so use that to your advantage. Try to experience the different sensations that can be aroused by a man and by a woman. It's guaranteed that they will each be able to arouse new pleasure that you've never felt before.

Two Men, One Woman

Another common form of the threesome, Two Men and One Woman is usually the fantasy for women. This can also be great for the men to experience penetration if they haven't already done so. Just like the previous threesome, this one is great for two people to focus on one. By doing this, you're able to give them a mixture of sensations that they wouldn't normally experience with just one partner. So, for example, both men can pleasure the woman's breasts while performing cunnilingus. Or, one can perform cunnilingus while the woman performs fellatio on the other. The most common position associated with this threesome is The Eiffel Tower. This is performed by having the woman go onto all fours while one man kneels behind her and the other in front. The man behind penetrates her while she performs fellatio to the man in the front. For an added effect the men can lean forward and clasp their hands together, mimicking the Eiffel Tower. This threesome is also good for experiencing double penetration which means one man inserts his penis into the woman's anus while the other inserts his penis into her vagina. Not only is this a really intense experience for the woman but because the holes are so close together, it makes the sensations around the penis very tight.

As you can tell, these threesomes are a great way to really mix up your sex life. There are many different things/positions you can try out that can enhance the sensations you feel. There's no wrong way to do it. You just need to start out slowly and feel your way around your partners. Group sex is also a great way for you to understand your partner's body more. By realizing that everyone has different ways of being pleasured, you'll be able to expand your knowledge of how to make your partner feel amazing in bed. Try out different techniques and experiment with toys or role play. Your sex life will become amazing in no time!

Chapter 7: Phone and Internet Sex

Sometimes couples end up being separated for a significant amount of time because of school or work. During this time, they aren't able to have intercourse except for the few visits that they pay each other during the time apart. This can put a strain on the relationship and many relationships don't survive long-distance. But technology has made it possible for people to feel close to each other even if they are thousands of miles away. Long-distance couples may not be able to experience their partner's touch but they can have a form of sexual intercourse through the phone and computer. This has even branched out to give those, who have trouble seeking out women or men, the ability to have a sexual connection with someone else. Phone and internet sex shouldn't be considered taboo or something weird, but rather as a way to bridge the gap in sexual experiences.

Phone Sex

Phone sex is great for couples that are in a long-distance relationship or simply can't get enough of each other. The wonderful thing about phone sex is that it leaves everything up to the imagination. You have to use your voice to "turn on" your partner on the other end. Generally, when you are having phone sex either you, your partner or both of you are masturbating. This is to help simulate the experience of actually having intercourse. Here are some tips on how to have really great phone sex.

- Let yourself go and try to stop being self-conscious. If this is your first time having phone sex you may feel a bit awkward in the beginning but just try to go with the flow. Once you and your partner get into it you won't even notice there's a phone between you.
- Try to set aside a time to have phone sex. It can be spontaneous but by setting a date and time, you can make sure that nothing interrupts you. This can also help both of you prepare if it's your first time.

- Get yourself ready. Even though your partner won't be able to see you, it can help you get in the mood if you feel sexier. Try setting up the bedroom as if your partner would be home. Light some candles, put on some music, dress yourself in some sexy lingerie, etc. It can also help if you start lightly touching yourself all over before you call each other. That way you're already hot and heavy. This also helps reduce nerves that can spring up when you actually perform the act.

- Make the call lighthearted. Remember that it's ok to have fun with this. Phone sex (and actual sex) doesn't have to be done in a correct way. You can start of the call with simply chatting about your day and working your way up to sex. Start talking about what you're doing in that moment, what you're wearing, how much you miss their touch, etc. to move the conversation towards sex. Try lowering your voice and/or your breathing to set a steamier mood.

- Really get descriptive with your sexy talk. Phone sex is all about imagination so you should try to get as descriptive as possible. Start by telling your partner what you're doing. For instance, let them know how wet you are or how hard you are. Asking them what to do is also a good way to escalate things. For example: "Should I remove my underwear?" "Where do you want me to touch next?" At the same time, you should also tell your partner what you want them to do. Let them know what you're imagining. This could be anything from a role play to something you two did in the past. You can tell them how much you want to kiss them on the mouth, how much you miss sex in the shower, etc. You can get as explicit as you want but generally, the more explicit the better. Remember to let them know how you're feeling. You can either describe how hot and horny you are for them or you can even moan. Start by just breathing heavier and work your way to louder moans.

- If you and your partner are masturbating, use these tips to help each other reach an orgasm. You might not always orgasm together so remember to keep the sexy talk going until they do. If one or both of you can't orgasm don't worry about it. Think of it as a build up to when you actually see each other.

- Try bringing in role play and toys into your phone sex session. It can make the talk more hot and heavy but it can also help you loosen up. By pretending to be someone else you can get over your fear of seeming ridiculous. Toys are also a great way to excite your partner and help stimulate you more. They also help relax you and make your breathing/moaning more loud and natural.

Phone sex can be very intimate which is why it's a great way for you and your partner to feel closer than ever, even when you're far apart. It requires a good amount of trust so you can feel comfortable that your partner won't laugh at you. Once you get past the awkward beginning, your imagination can lead you to places you've never even thought about. It can also help you become more open to other forms or fantasies of sex. Remember that good phone sex is a back and forth. Each of you needs to participate and add to the sexy talk. If only one of you is providing the details, then it won't feel as satisfying. Take this tips as a starting point for opening yourselves up to phone sex. Soon enough, you'll be naturals!

Tip: If you're really comfortable with phone sex try calling your partner at work (or somewhere risky) and use sexy talk to get them aroused in a public place. This is great for creating sexual tension that can be released with some really great sex at home!

As mentioned before, phone sex can also be conducted with strangers. There are specific organizations that employ people to offer this services and all you need is a phone number. By having phone sex with a stranger there's less pressure to "perform" perfectly. The employees are also trained so they can lead the conversation and help you to open up more. These tips can also work in this situation. It's also important to remember that there's no shame in calling these numbers. They can be a great way for people who have trouble meeting others to experience a form of sexual experience.

Internet Sex

Increasing technological advancements has really opened up the world of sex. Nowadays almost everyone has a computer/laptop and access to internet. Through this, couples and even single people now have the ability to enhance their sexual experience through sight. Like phone sex, internet sex is used to simulate sex through a medium. The difference between the two is that internet sex allows you to see your partner while a phone relies solely on voice. Being able to see your partner really enhances the sexual experience and can even be less nerve-wracking than phone sex. Here are some ways to get the most out of your online sexual experience.

- Get an account for video chatting. If you are planning on having internet sex with your partner it would be easiest if you both had a good way to internet chat. (This isn't necessary if you're going to be doing it with a stranger. There are sites specifically for this.) Make sure the service you choose has good quality and that your internet connection has fast speed. (You don't want your partner to freeze in the middle of the climax.)
- Set a time and date. This is really important so that nothing interrupts you. You don't want someone to bust in on you while your engaging in internet sex. It would also be good if you turned off any alarms or phones so that you don't get any rude interruptions. This also helps you prepare yourself if you're new to the experience. You can practice what you're going to say and do, and try to think of things to incorporate that might make the experience even better.
- Loosen up. Like phone sex, internet sex can seem very foreign and nerve wracking. It's important to remember that this is just another fun way of experiencing sex with your partner. It should help that you and your partner can see each other, adding to each of your sexual stimulation.

- Talk dirty to me. Although you can see each other there's still the downfall of not being able to touch each other. You both need to make up for this with some fun flirty, dirty talk. You can start of with simple conversation to help ease your way into the naughtier stuff. Simply steer the conversation towards how much you miss each other and how you can wait to touch them again. That should get things rolling.

- Get yourself ready. Because you can see each other it's a plus if you each put look sexier with a little outfit (or go nude). You can also set up your room with dim lights, music, candles, etc. Anything that can enhance your visualization of each other. You have the ability to look at each other with internet sex, so really use this to your advantage.

- Touch yourself. While you might feel strange masturbating on camera, it really adds to the sexual experience. Try getting into different positions. For example, if you're a woman, instead of facing the camera with your legs spread, turn around so that you're on all fours with you buttocks facing the camera. This is a really great angle that shows off your vagina and your butt. (It really turns on the men!)

- Get freaky with it. Internet sex is a great way to try out some of your more extreme fantasies before you actually perform them in the bedroom. Try proposing a certain role play to your partner and then both of you can try acting it out. It may turn out to be not as great as you thought or it might be seriously stimulating. (Which means it'll be even hotter in the bedroom.)

- Use toys. Since you have the benefit of being able to see each other, this is a great chance to use some toys. Vibrators and dildos are great for pleasuring yourself and helping your partner's imagination. But you can also use other things like a blindfold, nipple clamps or even a cock ring. This works well for masturbation but if you want to take it to the next level, mix it up with some role play.

Tip: If both you and your partner are really comfortable with having internet sex, set a date and time for it and start a role play as soon as you see each other. You can pretend your strangers having sex on the internet and make it a recurring thing that you do at a certain time and date. Try only doing it once a week so you each build up suspense and excitement. This also gives you a chance to thing of new things to add to the experience.

Internet sex can seem really strange at first but once you get into it, it's the next best thing to actually having sex with your partner. Depending on your own personal tastes, it can be harder for you to perform if your partner can see you but generally, this should help elevate the experience. Don't take it too seriously. There's no need to think you have to do what professionals do. Try new things and have fun with it but remember not to pressure you or your partner into doing anything you/they don't want to do. Internet sex is a great way to bridge distance in relationships and it can really open you up to learning more about your partner and yourself.

Chapter 8: Swingers Clubs

If you and your partner feel like you've experienced all there is to experience with sex, think again. Swingers clubs offer couples the chance to switch partners for a night of sex with someone new.

Trust is the most important thing you need to remember when swinging. You need to be sure that this is something both of you want to do and that neither of you consider it cheating. There also needs to be trust between you and your swinging partner. Many swingers find each other on the internet because their lifestyle is considered too taboo to openly talk about. So, if you and your partner find others to swing with, be honest about who you are, what you look like, etc. You're going to share a very intimate experience with a stranger so you need to be open and honest. Discuss what you and your partner want out of this experience. One of you might be looking for something sensual while the other is looking for more of BDSM.

Once you've settled on what you both want you need to decide if you're going to go to a club or simply find an open couple. If you want to find a couple your best bet is to look on the internet. (If you do meet a couple from the internet, make sure you meet them first before you invite them into their home.) Many times people post fake accounts which can put you and your partner in danger. By meeting them in a public space you can get to know them a little better to see if they are dangerous or not. It can be awkward to meet a couple from the internet so try to make the meeting place somewhere fun like a bar. It's good to know if they are compatible with you or not in person. If you both feel like you've hit off, then invite them to your place and start swinging!

Clubs or parties are generally the place to go first if you're a beginner. Not only does it feel much safer but you can see how more experienced swingers act. It's important to remember that if you go to a club you don't have to participate in any sexual activity if you don't want to. You can go to observe which is one of the best ways to learn how to swing. It's also a great way to meet different people and find couples to swing with regularly. The clubs vary from place to place so there's always something new to experience. They generally have different themed rooms that allow the couples to try out different activities. For example, one room might contain toys that you're suppose to use on each other and another might be a dark room that encourages partners to touch each other without knowing who's who.

Because the experience of swinging is such an intimate act performed with strangers there are rules and codes. We've listed some general rules to follow at swinging clubs. (Different clubs have different rules so find out what they are before you go.)

- Make sure you set up rules for yourself that you communicate to other swingers. If you are against using toys make that known. That way you don't waste yours and other peoples time. It will also help you keep from getting into a situation where you don't want to be.
- Ask. If you see a couple that you want to join, ask them first before jumping in. They may already be getting hot and heavy and don't need anyone else or they might be looking for another person to help spice things up. If they look like they're about to climax, wait until they're done and then approach them.
- Present yourself. Don't be afraid to go all out and dress yourself up. The product your selling here is yourself so make yourself irresistible. Wear the sexiest lingerie you own or the fanciest suit that makes you looking dashing. You want everyone's head to turn when you walk into the club.
- Get to know each other. If you find a couple that you like you don't have to immediately go into a playroom. Most clubs offer food and drinks so take a seat and start by telling them a little about yourself and vice versa. It's much

easier to get naked in front of strangers when you learn more about them and you feel like you know them.

- Be safe. Bring condoms if you're a man and make sure the man wears a condom if you're a woman. Just because someone's at a swingers' club doesn't mean they're disease free. You could easily catch something you don't want. You also want to avoid getting anyone or yourself pregnant.
- Privacy agreement. Some clubs, if not all, will make you sign a non-disclosure agreement which says that you agree not to tell anyone what goes on at the club. But this also goes for the people. You should never speak about the couples you swing with as they might be keeping it a secret. It is up to you if you wish to tell anyone that you participate in this lifestyle but the identities of your partners should remain private out of respect for them.
- Some clubs have different ways of mixing up people. For instance, one club might use a colored wristband and tell certain colors to talk to others. This helps make sure things are fair and also allows people to meet someone they might not necessarily talk to first. It's also good for helping beginners get over their nervousness and meeting some people.

Swingers clubs aren't for everybody but they are definitely worth trying out if you and your partner are open to it. Go to a club first if you're nervous about participating and simply watch. It may end up turning you on and help your decision on whether to join or not. Remember that you are always in control of what happens and if you are uncomfortable you can always say no. Swinging is a really rewarding sexual experience that most people end up coming back for.

Chapter 9: Sex While Pregnant

When pregnant women get a rush of different hormones that make their moods kind of erratic. One of the hormones that gets increased is estrogen and progesterone. This increases their libido and makes them really horny. Now, many people think that having sex while pregnant can actually hurt the baby. This is not true. The penis cannot go past the vagina which means the baby is perfectly safe while momma gets it on. Some positions are safer than others and help increase the sensations felt. We've listed the top 5 positions for the best sex while pregnant.

Remember to only have sex as long as your pregnancy is normal. It's common that women experience bleeding during intercourse so don't be worried if this happens to you. Make sure you mention it to your doctor so they can check that everything is fine with you and the baby. Having sex near the due date can also help induce labor. **Warning:** If you're partner goes down on you, make sure they don't blow air into your vagina. This could cause an air bubble to block one of your blood vessels and hurt the baby.

The Spoon

The Spoon is a great move that doesn't really require much movement. It's also one of the more comfortable positions for the woman. Start out by lying on your side and then have your man lie behind you. Arch your back so that your buttocks stick into his crotch. Then, have him insert his penis into your vagina. When you're comfortable he can begin thrusting slowly. It's always best to start out slowly so you can get use to the sensation and make sure that nothing is hurting. If you want, you can also control the thrusting by moving your hips back and forth. The further away your bodies are bigger the range of movement. Although, this move is good for slow penetration and it also stops his penis from going so deep. That doesn't mean to say it isn't good for him. Your closed legs put more pressure on his penis making your vagina feel tighter, which is great for him.

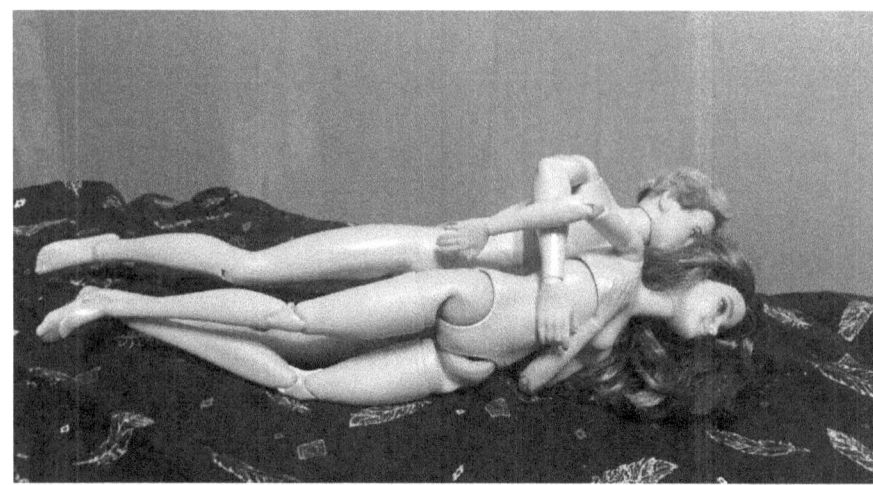

Picture 55 Sex While Pregnant The Spoon

Ride 'em Cowgirl

Ride 'em Cowgirl is the traditional sex pose where the woman is on top. This pose is especially good for pregnant women because it allows them to control the depth of penetration and the speed. Start by having your man lie on his back, then climb on top of him so that your legs are on either side of his hips. Lower yourself on his penis slowly. This way you can gauge just how deep you want his penis to penetrate. Lift your hips up and down to start thrusting. You can also move your hips back and forth to rub his penis on the inside of your vagina. Make sure to do whatever feels good to you. Pregnancy can sometimes make you feel less sexy so try putting on a show. Play with your breasts and nipples. When you see your man getting hot for you it'll turn you on even more.

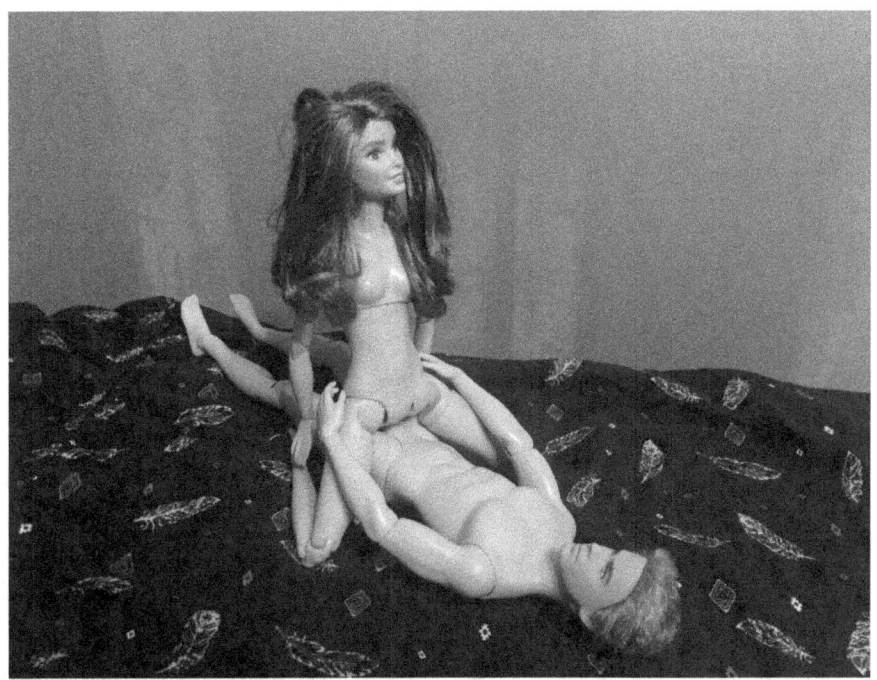

Picture 56 Sex While Pregnant Ride 'em Cowgirl

Superman

The Superman is another spin on the traditional pose, missionary. It's hard to perform the missionary pose while pregnant because of the danger of squishing the baby. Fortunately, there is a variation to this pose that doesn't require the man to lie on top of you but you still get all the benefits of the pose. Start by lying on your back with your feet up and at the edge of the bed. Then have your man come stand between your legs and slowly insert his penis into your vagina. You can choose to put your legs down, keep them up or even wrap them around his waist if you are able to. Then have him place his hands on the bed next to you so that he can hover over you without putting his weight on the baby. He can also place his hands on your hips or your legs if he prefers. Then, while standing he can start thrusting slowly. Try voicing what you want him to do, for instance, if you want him to go faster. Chances are he's going to be really gentle with you unless you tell him otherwise.

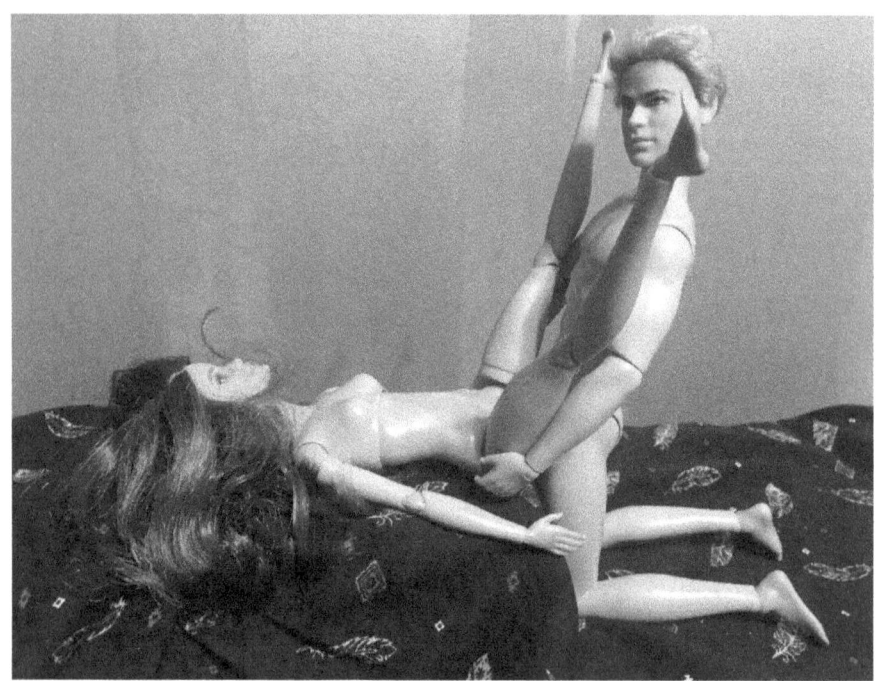

Picture 57 Sex While Pregnant Ride 'em Cowgirl

Couch Potato

This move is a variation on the traditional doggy style. Generally, it's a pretty uncomfortable pose and sometimes hard for women to even get into at all. This variation is a lot easier. Start by kneeling on the bed or a couch and bending over slightly so your back is at a 45-degree angle. You can rest your hands on the arm rest or your thighs for balance. Then have your man come kneel behind you. When you feel stable have him insert his penis from behind. He can hold your hips or your shoulders to balance both of you. Then he can begin thrusting. This pose allows his penis to go pretty deep so make sure he starts out slowly so you can adjust yourself. If it begins to hurt have him stop immediately and then decide if you want to try it again in that pose or continue with something else.

Take a Seat is a really easy move to perform that feels great. Have your man sit on the edge of the bed or in a chair. Then, while either facing him or with your back towards him slowly sit down on his lap while you insert his penis into your vagina. This pose is felt more deeply if your back is facing him so take that into consideration when you perform this move. You have control over the depth of penetration and the speed which is what makes this such a great pose for pregnant women. Unlike Ride em' Cowboy you also have better control and range of motion because of the position you are in. It can help if you have something to hold onto so you can lift yourself up and down to increase thrusting speed. This pose can also get very tiring for the legs but if you have something to hold onto, the legs don't have to work as hard.

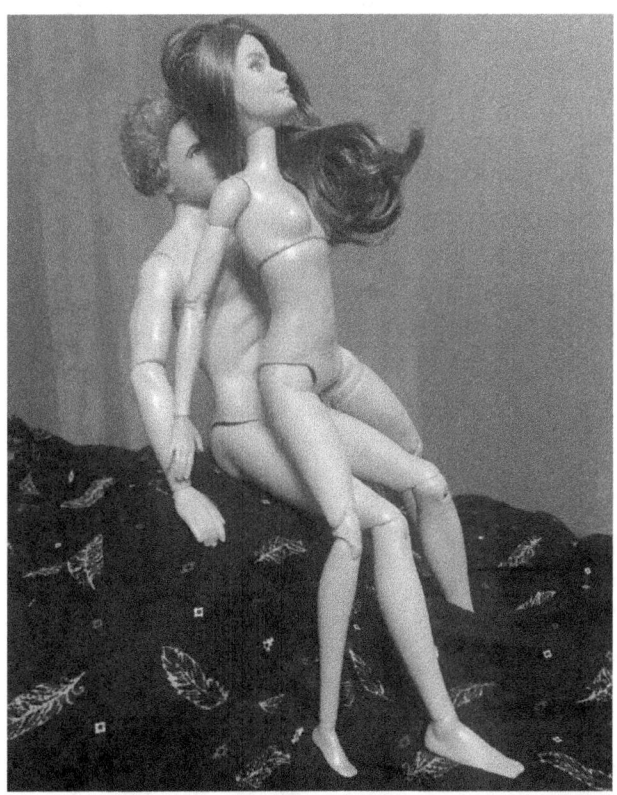

Picture 58 Sex While Pregnant Take a Seat

Tip: Since your positions can be limited while pregnant this is a good chance to try out other types of sexual interactions. For instance, role playing can help enhance the position that you are choosing. Or you can also try using toys like a blindfold or even a clit stimulator. For men things like cock rings can magic wands can also bring an added amount of pleasure.

These positions give you the best range of motion and hit the spot just right. During your second and third trimester it's best if you refrain from positions that have you lying flat on your back. It puts pressure on your aorta which cuts off blood flow to the placenta. If you want to do a position that requires you to lay on your back, place a pillow underneath your left hip. This keeps the baby from putting pressure on the aorta.

Pregnancy doesn't have to stop you from enjoying the benefits of sex. Just remember to use caution so nothing happens to you or the baby. If you're nervous about doing it for the first time, talk about it with your doctor. They can give you a checkup and let you know if it's safe to have sex. If anytime during sex you feel discomfort or pain, stop. Let your doctor know what happened and then proceed from there. Most of the time it won't be anything serious but it's better to be safe. And as always, have fun with it!

Part III: Aftertaste

Chapter 10: Techniques of Erotic Massage

Erotic massage is a technique used to stimulate a person's erogenous zones and get the body's circulation going. Not only does it feel amazing, but it helps to sexually arouse your partner. It can be used before sex to help stimulate each other or it can be done after sex, for further relaxation. Here are some tips on how to stimulate your partner with a simple massage.

- Set the mood. The massage is supposed to be erotic so make sure the environment works to create a sensual mood. Put on some soft, slow music, light some candles, etc. Make sure the place your partner lies down on is firm and stable.
- Make sure you have some oil. Lotion works as well but oil is more slippery and doesn't absorb as fast as oil. Some good options are coconut, avocado, grapeseed and jojoba. The oil helps make the skin more slippery so your hands can slide around smoothly. Plus, it's also great for making your skin look healthy.
- There are several different techniques you can use for your massage: shiatsu, compression, stroking, friction and kneading.
  - Shiatsu is done by laying your hands or fingers on a specific spot and applying pressure while slowly rotating. This technique is great for working out some really deep knots. Remember to start with a soft pressure and work your way to a deeper one. If you are more experienced with this technique you can use your elbow to apply so really hard pressure.
  - Compression is done by pressing down on one specific area. This increases blood flow and loosens the muscles. It's a good technique to use on areas around the spine and the shoulder blades. You can use it as a beginning more to warm up the body or an ending move to get rid of any tension still left.

o   Stroking is comprised of long gentle movements all along the body. Keep your fingers together and place your whole hand on your partner's body. Then slowly run your hands up and down their back, legs and arms. It is a very gentle move that helps you get acquainted with the feel of their body. It is also very slow and hypnotic for the person receiving the massage. You can try applying different types of pressure to enhance the pleasure.

o   Friction is generally used without oils but it feels good both ways. This technique focuses on small specific areas on the body and is great for the hands and feet. It is performed by taking an area of the body between the thumbs and index finger (or any other finger) and rubbing in a circular motion. It's great for working out really hard knots and for relaxing tougher areas of the body.

o   Kneading is great for the fleshier parts of the body, such as the buttocks. It's also used to get really deep into the muscles. You can use different types of pressure with this move depending on how your partner likes it. Take a part of the body and grasp it firmly in your hand. Then lift it up and press down on it with the palm of your hand. Do this all over in a rhythmic motion for the best results.

•   Warmth. Make sure all aspects of the massage are warm. You want your partner to achieve maximum relaxation. The room and the surface that your partner lies on should be warm. Turn up the heat and lay a blanket or towel down. You can also heat up the oil in the microwave or by rubbing it between your hands first. Make sure that your hands are also warm before you begin. You don't want to shock your partner with cold fingers.

•   Keep the connection. Once you start massaging your partner, make sure one of your hands is always touching them. It helps maintain the sensual connection that you've been building up through touch. If you need to do something, like apply more oil, keep one hand on the body while the other gets the oil. This is why it's good to have all the things you'll need for the massage within reaching distance.

Now that you've learned the setup, we've listed some areas that will make your partner melt in your hands. Remember that these are just suggestions. If you or your partner wish to massage other areas, go for it! Erotic massage is all about feeling each other's bodies and learning to read their sexual language.

Face

Take your index and middle finger, on both hands, and slowly press into the side of your partner's temples. Release and gently press again. You can also move your fingers in small circular motions while you press down. Then gently slide your fingers down the sides of his cheeks either in a straight line or while you continue making small circular motions. Lightly trace your fingers around his lips and his jaw. The outer edges of the lips actually have a lot of sensory neurons that can be stimulated with small movements and light touches. Tell your partner to close their eyes for an added effect. You can also take your fingers and lightly drag them all across their face. This is highly stimulating because it feels great and they don't know where you are going to touch them next.

Neck

The neck actually contains a gland that regulates body functions, such as sex drive. The front of the neck is especially sensitive to any touches. Use your hand to stroke your partner's neck while you kiss them. Cup your hand and pull at the back of the neck to convey your desire. You can also use your mouth to lightly breath across the skin and kiss/bite. Some of the most sensitive areas of the neck include the base where it meets the shoulder, the hollow between the neck and the chest and for men, the Adam's apple. As you are kissing the neck, try massaging the shoulders at the same time. This way you are relaxing them, as you are arousing them.

Ears

Ears are a really big erogenous zone that often get overlooked. They may be small but they are packed with lots of tiny nerve endings that can really work you up. Take the earlobes into both of your hands and gently squeeze with you thumb and index finger. Rub them between your fingers with a circular motion and slowly pull down. Do this to the whole ear, not just the earlobe. Even though the earlobe is the fleshiest part of the ear, this technique feels good on the whole thing. To turn up the erotic factor, try licking around the earlobe. Then slowly suck it into your mouth and nibble on it for a few seconds. You can also kiss the area behind the ear, as this is another sensitive area.

Hands

Our hands do a lot of things throughout the day that we don't really take notice of. Massaging them is a great way to help them relax and it can be even feel sensual. There's a reason couples hold hands. Start by taking your partner's hand between yours. Using your fingers, gently press into the palm and move in a circular motion. Do this to the center of the palm but also around the outer edge of the whole hand. Take your thumb and index and squeeze on the webbed part between the fingers. You can also lightly drag your fingers along the outer edge of the hand, beside the thumb and pinky. Hands are actually pretty sensitive so applying different pressures to different parts can be quite a pleasurable experience.

Lower Back

The kidneys have often been thought to be the source of sex drive. They're located along the lower back, above the waist and if massaged properly it can create much more than a relaxed feeling. Start at the sacrum (the triangular bone at the base of the spine, also known as the tailbone). It has little holes that contain lots of nerve endings guaranteed to wake up the pelvis. Place your palm flat on top of the sacrum and gently push down, slowly building up pressure. Then start kneading into it to create heat that will warm up skin and stimulate the groin. Take your thumbs and press into the area above the hips, near the base of the spine. The lower back works hard to keep the rest of the body up so use a lot of pressure to relax the muscles and loosen up the lower body.

Stomach

The stomach is never really thought of as an erogenous zone, but it is. The area between the navel and lower stomach (happy trail) is especially sensitive for the man. This is because of its connection to the perineum, the erogenous zone behind his balls. Take your fingers and lightly press down from the naval to the base of the penis or the top of the vagina. The area around the belly button is also very sensitive. Using your fingertips, slowly create circles around the belly button that get bigger as you move towards the outside of the abdomen. Remember to apply a good amount of pressure without hurting your partner, otherwise you could end up just tickling them.

Thighs

The thighs, especially around the crotch, build up a lot of pressure throughout the day that never really gets relaxed. If you've ever stretched out those areas, you'll know just how amazing it feels to work out that built up tension. It's also a highly erogenous zone because of its proximity to the genitals. Take your hands and with a medium amount of pressure, squeeze the thighs. Work from the knees up towards the genitals. When you get to the top of the thighs, take your thumbs and press on the triangular area where the legs meet the hips. This area can get very tight so start lightly and slowly build up the pressure. Press in circular motions around the hips, all the way to the buttocks. You can also squeeze the butt quite hard for added pleasure. Try to avoid touching the genitals so you can focus on the areas the don't get much attention, but also create some sexual tension.

Feet

In Chinese medicine, the feet contain healing points for all parts of the body. When they are stimulated, through massage or acupuncture, specific areas of the body are invigorated that help it to heal. This also works as an erogenous zone which can help relax the body and stimulate the groin. Take your hand and make it into a fist. Press your knuckles into the heel of the foot, working your way up to the base of the toes. Then, with your fingers, rub the whole foot in circular, pressing motions. Use a strong pressure in this area to avoid ticking. You can also try pulling the toes with a sharp jerk. It releases pressure between the joints and can even crack the toes. To make it even more erotic, you can kiss the foot and even suck on the toes.

Everyone's body is different so if you are getting the massage, make sure you communicate with your partner what you do and don't like. You can also throw in some sexy moans and body movements to let them know that you are enjoying what they're doing. It will also make them feel good, that they are able to pleasure you so much. At the same time, remember not to talk to much. Erotic massage is about feeling each other and learning to communicate through touch. Once you've settled in, close your eyes, and relax into the feeling of your partner's hands running all over your body.

Chapter 11: Tantric Sex

Tantric sex is an ancient Eastern spiritual practice meant to expand consciousness and join the masculine and feminine energy into one. In Sanskrit, the word Tantra means, "woven together". It uses rituals that enable people to enjoy sex more often and for longer periods of time. Not only does it increase your sexual energy, it also stimulates your physical, mental and emotional capacities. It goes beyond the bedroom and into all aspects of life. Tantric sex teaches you how to be present in all moments and experience everything fully. It is not your everyday sexual experience. It is a deep sexual experience that requires an open mind and the right information. The key to good Tantra is found in the breath. Through meditation and focused breath you can spread sexual and orgasmic energy from your genitals to your whole body. We've listed some tips on how to enter into a Tantric sex experience.

- Make your space. Tantric sex is a process that takes time. Prepare your bed or wherever you plan to do it, with lots of pillows and blankets. Have lots of candles around the area and either dim the lights or turn them off completely. Make sure you have water or light wine that you can reach throughout the session. You can also have food nearby to feed each other, such as grapes or strawberries.
- Minimize distractions. Turn of your phones and alarms so that nothing disturbs you during this time. Make sure that you don't have any pressing appointments or anything to do. This way you can forget about the future and the past and focus completely on the present.
- Prepare yourself. You need to have an open mind when you enter into this experience. If anything makes you uncomfortable you can choose not to do it, but try to get past your feeling of discomfort. This is usually brought on by the feelings of shame and in tantric sex there is no shame between you and your partner. The whole experience should be open and playful. Wear comfortable clothes, like underwear or you can choose to be nude.

- Build the sexual energy. Start by facing each other and stretching to release any tension. Then either sit cross-legged in front of each other or place your legs on top of each other so that your genitals are facing. Begin by looking into each other's eyes for a long time. It will be uncomfortable at first but over time it will seem natural. Keep maintaining eye contact until it feels comfortable. This is when you know the connection has been established. Try to maintain this eye contact throughout the whole Tantra session.
- Follow these steps:
  - Breathe together. Steady your breathing so that both of you inhale and exhale simultaneously. Make sure you are still looking into each other's eyes. You can also put your hands on each other's chest to feel the breath entering and exiting, as well as the heartbeat.
  - When you are synchronized, say some things to your partner that will connect you further. For example: "I love when you __." Your statements should be truthful and should reflect exactly how you feel about your partner. Take turns sharing your thoughts.
  - Take your fingertips and slowly move them across your partner's body. This will wake up the nerves and heighten the sensations felt. Move your hands close to your partner's genitals and breasts but don't touch them.
  - Move into the Yab-Yum position, where the man is sitting cross-legged and the woman sits on top, facing him. Hug each other and breathe together while in this position.
  - Begin some tantric kissing. Keep your lips slightly open while they touch and breathe together in the same synchronized manner. Feel how you share the same breath. Then join your lips in a soft, sensual kiss.
  - Give each other a tantric massage. Start by massaging the non-erogenous zones and then slowly move to those areas. You can utilize techniques from the erotic massage during this stage. However, this massage is not focused on sexual stimulation so do not try to arouse them or bring them to orgasm.
  - Consummate your love. Sex is not the focus of Tantra but one of the options. You can also choose to end the

session by lying together in a relaxed state. If you do have sex, move slowly. Choose a position that enhances the connection you feel with your partner and one that preferably allows you to maintain eye contact. Make sure you stay focused in the moment so that you can feel the energy and connection between you and your partner building up to the climax.

    o   After orgasm, stay in the same position until your breathing and heart rate return back to normal. Look into each other's eyes and stroke each other's faces. Then slowly disconnect from each other. If you want the connection to remain you can lie down next to each other or have the woman lie on top of the man.

    o   Finishing. Tantric sexual philosophy believes that the physical union between humans is sacred and therefore it should be treated as such. When your body's have returned to normal sit facing each with your knees touching. Put your right hand, palm up on each other's left knee and close your eyes. Feel the connection slowly starting to leave your bodies. When you feel it has gone, move so that you are sitting in your own space. Open your eyes when you are ready and give thanks for the experience that you have shared.

•   Practice. Tantric sex requires lots of practice. You learn to be one with your partner but also with yourself. The first couple of times that you engage in Tantra it will feel strange and possibly a little awkward. But if you keep at it, you will learn how to move with your partner as one. Not only is it great for enhancing your sexual experience, it brings you closer to your partner in all aspects of life.

One of the most important goals of tantric sex is learning to keep the energy that would normally leave your body during an orgasm. The art of Tantra teaches you to prolong the sexual act and your orgasm so that you can increase your sexual energy and the intimacy between you and your partner. It takes the act of sex and turns it into a means for transformation rather than a simple act of recreation. There is no goal in Tantra which makes the act of sex more intimate, expressive and even meditative. Women and even men have experienced prolonged multiple orgasm in one Tantra session.

If you're just starting out with Tantra, try spending several week practicing without engaging in intercourse. This will really help you learn to build a connection and it can also show you that you can experience intimacy without having to touch each other. It's also a good way to experience other intense emotions or feelings that come along with sex but that can be hidden by the strength of an orgasm. If your love life has gone a little stale, Tantra is great for reawakening intimate emotions and building trust with your partner.

Remember that Tantric sex isn't about having sex for an extended period of time, although that is usually an effect. But really Tantra, is about establishing a connection between you and your partner that you carry throughout the duration of your experience. In the beginning you might end up rushing to the part where you have intercourse and that's ok. Eventually, you will learn to experience all aspects of your partner and this is what will make sex feel more extended. You will learn to please your partner with your eyes, with your words and with your hands. And in the end you will move and feel as if you are one person.

When you feel more comfortable with Tantra, try exploring a sexual taboo together. For example, you can experiment with some bondage or even try a new position, like anal. By exploring a new area together, you become closer to each other through a shared experience. It also shows how much you trust each other. Sexual taboos tend to make people feel ashamed for participating in a strange sexual act. This keeps people from exploring different areas that can actually be quite pleasurable. Tantra allows you to open up to your partner so that both of you can face each other without shame. By engaging in a taboo sexual act together you are able to open yourself up to your partner completely and experience something truly wonderful.

Chapter 12: Sex and Yoga

Not only is yoga a great way to stretch and re-energize your body, many of the poses are fantastic for sex. The poses offer deeper penetration, better stimulation and they help build more intimacy between you and your partner. The key to yogic sex is breathing. It helps release the same chemicals in the brain that sex does. Certain poses are also great for increasing blood flow to the pelvis and creating sexual arousal. Some of the benefits of regular yoga practice include longer erections and longer orgasms.

There are hundreds of different yoga poses that range from beginner to more advanced. We've listed some poses to help you get started. If you practice yoga, this poses will be familiar to you and therefore, you can experiment more with your range of motion. If you don't practice yoga, some of this poses can be straining on the muscles, so start slowly and don't overexert yourself or you could cause injury. Make sure to warm up a little first before you attempt these poses during sex.

Child's Pose

This pose is very easy and can be performed by anyone, no matter what your flexibility level is. Make sure you have something soft on your knees so that they don't get sore or bruised. Start by kneeling on the ground with your legs together and then sitting back on your legs. You may need to adjust a little if your ankles are not flexible enough. If it's easier, you can also spread your knees apart so that only your toes are touching. When you are in a comfortable position, lower your head so that your torso is lying on your thighs and your head is touching the ground. Your arms can either be stretched in front of you or lying beside your legs. Have your man come up behind you and place his hands on your hips. You may need to lift your butt up for him to insert his penis but try to keep it as close to your feet as you can. This pose doesn't offer a lot of range of motion which makes it good for a slower, deeper sexual experience. The angle of your body causes the penis to hit a very sensitive spot in the vagina. It is also great for the man because your position makes the vagina very tight around his penis.

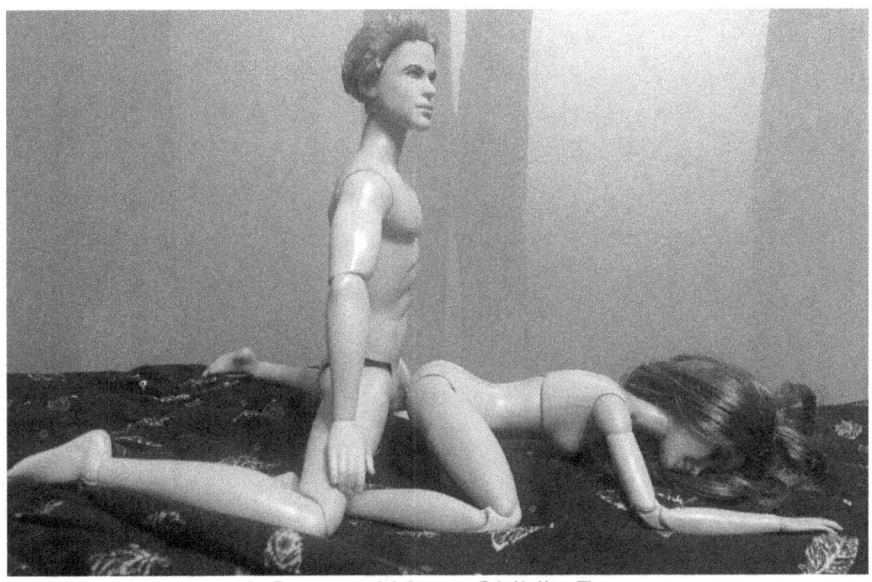

Picture 59 Sex and Yoga Child's Pose

Happy Baby

Happy Baby is a relatively easy pose but it can be straining on the hip muscles. Take some time to warm up the inner groin with a few light stretches, before getting into this pose. When you're ready, begin by lying on your back. Take your feet or your ankles into your hands so that your legs are at a 90-degree angle. Rock from side to side so that you get used to the feeling of the pose and so you can stretch out any tightness in your inner groin. When you are comfortable return to lying still on your back. Have your man position himself between your legs and slowly insert his penis into your vagina. He can either thrust from a kneeling position or if you are more flexible he can lie on top of you, like in missionary pose. This yoga pose is great for really getting in deep. By spreading your legs wide and angling your pelvis up, your vagina becomes more open. This allows his penis to go deeper and hit the G-spot more easily.

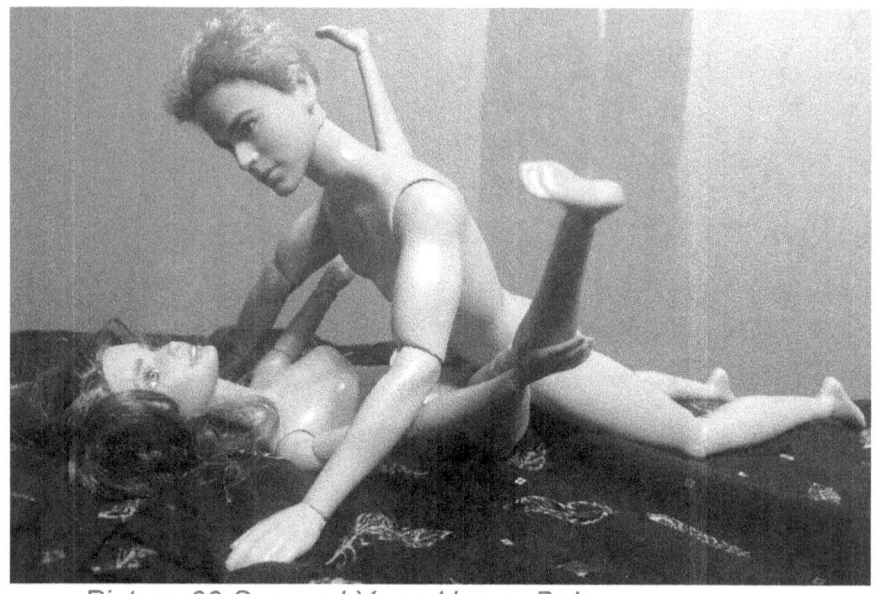

Picture 60 Sex and Yoga Happy Baby

Downward Dog

Downward Dog one of the most well-known poses in yoga. It does require some degree of stability and flexibility when used as sex pose. Start out on your hands and knees. Press into the ground with your hands as you extend you knees backward, raising your butt into the air. To make this pose easier, keep your knees slightly bent. If you have more flexibility you can straighten your legs and try to put your heels on the ground. Have your man stand behind you, with his legs on either side of yours. He may have to squat slightly to insert his penis into your vagina. If you are a really advanced yogi, you can lift one of your legs up so that it's resting against your man's chest. This pose has a lot of stability to you can thrust harder and faster.

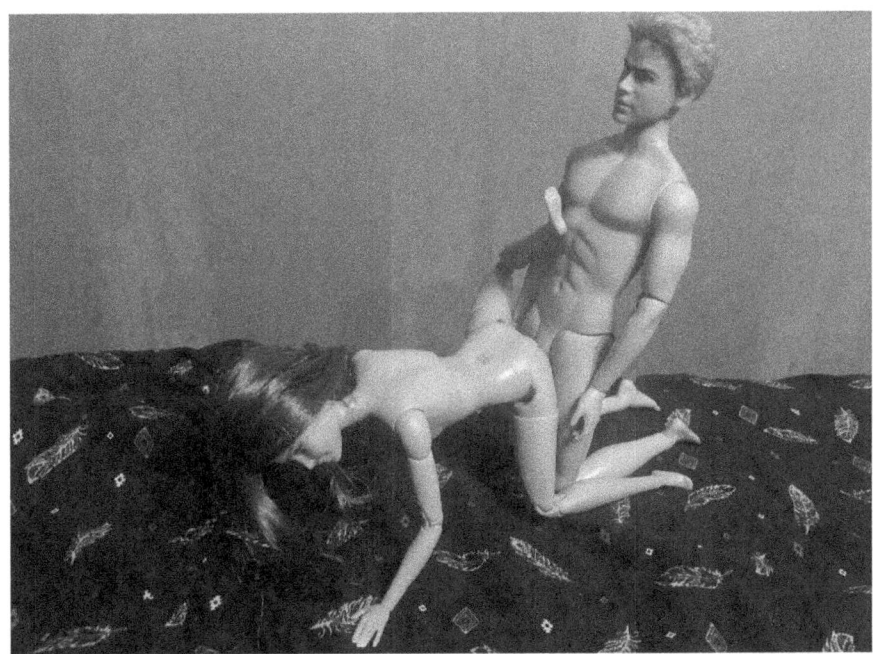

Picture 61 Sex and Yoga Downward Dog

Puppy Dog

The Puppy Dog is a slightly easier version of Downward Dog. Start by coming onto all fours, like you would in Downward Dog. This time lower your front completely so that your chest is as close to the ground as possible, while your butt remains in the air. This pose is a great stretch for the back and shoulders as well as an amazing sex position. Have your man come up behind you with his knees on either side on your legs. Adjust yourself, if necessary, so that he can insert his penis into your vagina. You can also choose to thrust if you are comfortable is this pose. Lift your chest up slightly so that it isn't touching the ground. You can rock yourself back and forth with your hands or, if you have more lower back flexibility, you can move your butt back and forth to create a thrusting motion.

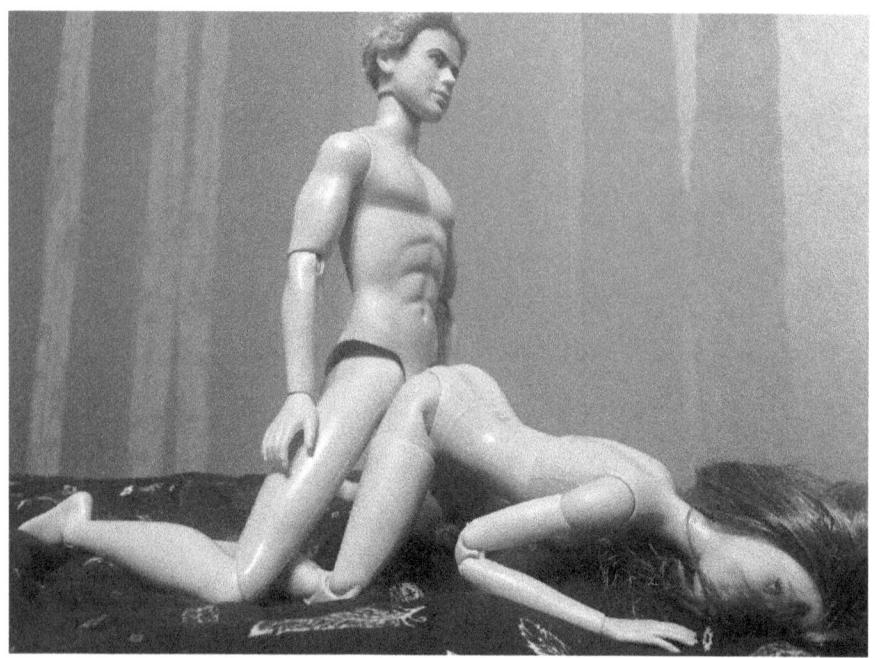

Picture 62 Sex and Yoga Puppy Dog

Reclined Pigeon

Reclined Pigeon is a simple pose that is great for stretching out the lower back and buttocks, and for hitting that elusive G-spot. Start by laying on your back with your feet flat on the floor and your knees bent. Then take one leg and cross it over the other so that your ankle is resting on your other thigh. Lift your upper body slightly so that you can slip one hand between your legs while you wrap the other around your thigh and clasp your hands together. When you lay back down your hands should lift your leg into the air and you should feel a stretch in the leg that is crossed. If you are more flexible you can always pull your leg closer to your chest. It may take a few seconds for your body to adjust to the stretch. When you are comfortable have your man kneel in front of you legs and insert his penis into your vagina and begin thrusting. This pose makes the vagina very tight but it also allows the penis to go deeper. If your arms get tired you can always let go of your thigh and have it rest against his chest. Depending on how flexible you are he can also push down as if he were lying on top of you. This deepens the sensations felt by both of you.

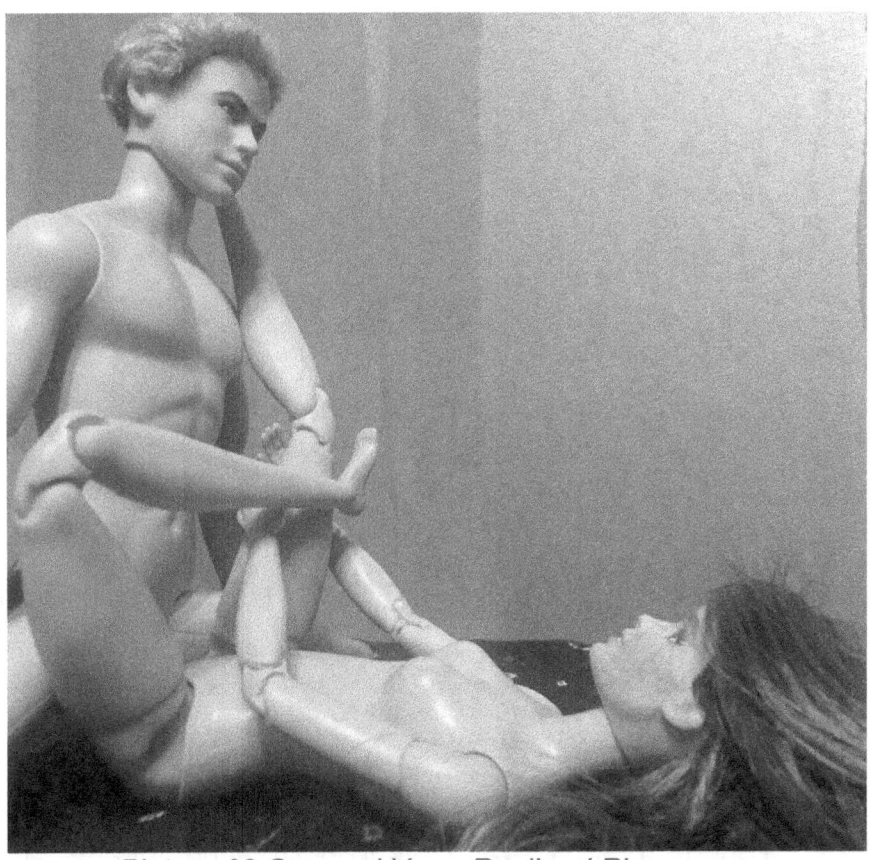

Picture 63 Sex and Yoga Reclined Pigeon

Straddle Forward Fold

This pose slightly advanced because of the amount of flexibility needed in the legs. Stand with your legs spread wide apart and your feet facing outwards. Then, hinge at the waist and lower yourself as far as you can go so that your hands touch the floor. If you can't go that low, you can also place your hands on your legs or on a wall for balance. Your man can then come up behind you and insert his penis into your vagina. The deeper you go in the fold, the more intense the sensations will be. If your hands are on the ground or he wall you can also take control of the thrusting. Try some different variations, such as going in circles or moving your hips up and down to create some friction.

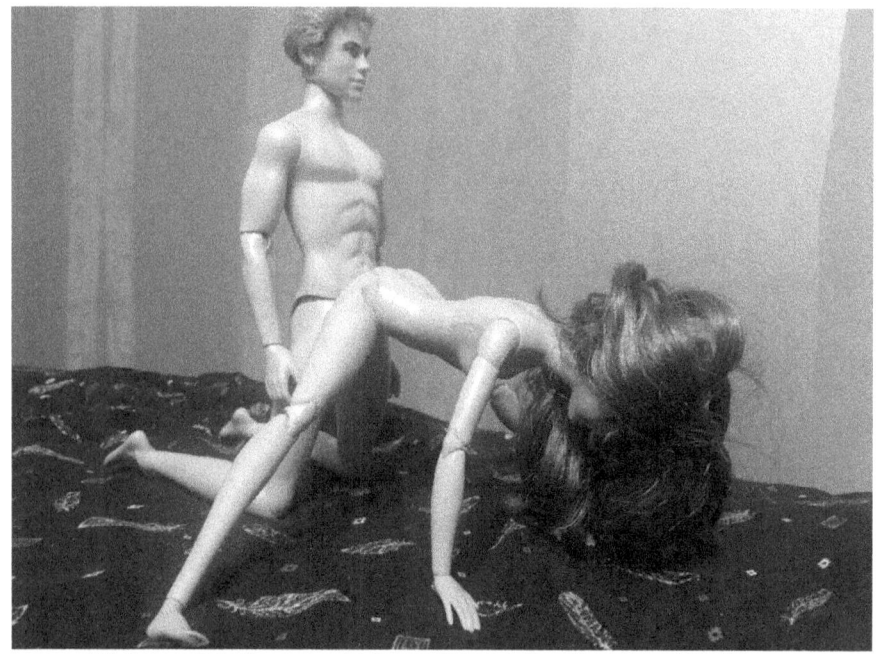

Picture 64 Sex and Yoga Straddle Forward Fold

Bridge
Bridge pose elevates your pelvis and creates an amazing angle for pleasurable sensations. To get into this pose, start by lying on your back with your feet, flat on the floor near your buttocks. Clasp your hands underneath your back and press into your feet and arms so that your pelvis moves up and your butt leaves the floor. Try to position yourself so that your upper body is resting on your shoulders and not your neck. Then, spread your legs apart so that your man can position himself between them and insert his penis. This pose restricts your movement so your man will be in control of thrusting. Make sure he doesn't go too hard or too fast as it could cause injury to your neck. For added pleasure, squeeze your legs together so that the pressure in your vagina

is increased. If you are both more advanced you can try wrapping your legs around his waist so that only your shoulders and head are on the ground.

Plow Pose

This pose really changes up the angle that the penis enters into the vagina. It's really great for experiencing new sensations and for hitting the G-spot. However, it is really hard on the neck so you may want to put something soft down. Start by lying flat on your back with your legs stretched out. Lift your legs and pelvis so that your legs are in the air. You can support your back with your hands if you need to. Then lower you legs so that your toes touch down behind your head. If you have more flexibility you can also lower your knees down so that they are beside your ears. Have your man come up behind you and stand so that he is almost on top of you. Then he can slowly lower himself down to insert his penis into your vagina. Depending on where he is standing this pose can be a variation of The Pile Driver. He can thrust as hard and as fast as he wants but make sure your neck is completely stability. If not, it can cause some serious damage. If you are new to yoga, for safety, start out slowly and work your way up.

Camel Pose

Camel pose in yogic sex is actually performed by the man which allows the woman to control more of the movement. Start by kneeling on a soft surface. Place your hands on your lower back and slowly hinge backwards so that you are looking up. Depending on your flexibility you might be able to place your hands on your ankles and do a half-backbend. This pose will thrust your penis forward. When you are comfortable your woman should place herself on all fours with her buttocks facing your penis. She can then back up so that your penis penetrates her vagina. This pose is great for both partners because it allows the woman to take control while the man can focus on the sensations. Because the penis is thrust forward it also allows it to go in much deeper than normal.

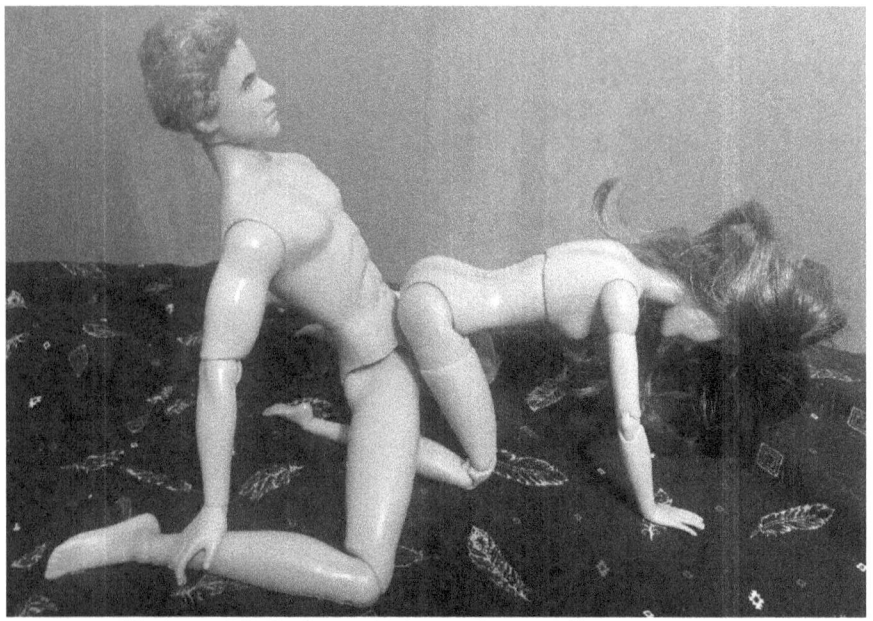

Picture 65 Sex and Yoga Camel Pose

Chair Pose

Chair pose is another one that puts the woman in control. This pose is advanced and requires a lot of muscle strength in both the man and the woman. Start by standing upright and tensing your leg muscles. Lift your arms above your head and slowly push your butt backwards, as if you were about to sit in a chair. Stop when your thighs are at a 45-degree angle. If this pose is too difficult, you can also use a wall to take some of the pressure off your legs. Then have your woman stand in front of you, with her back towards your face, and push her butt backwards so that your penis penetrates her vagina. Depending on her level of strength and flexibility, she can go into the same pose or she can do variations on the foreword fold. This pose restricts movement slightly but it puts the penis in the perfect angle to hit the G-spot. If neither of you can manage this pose you can also start by sitting on a chair and working your way up to the pose.

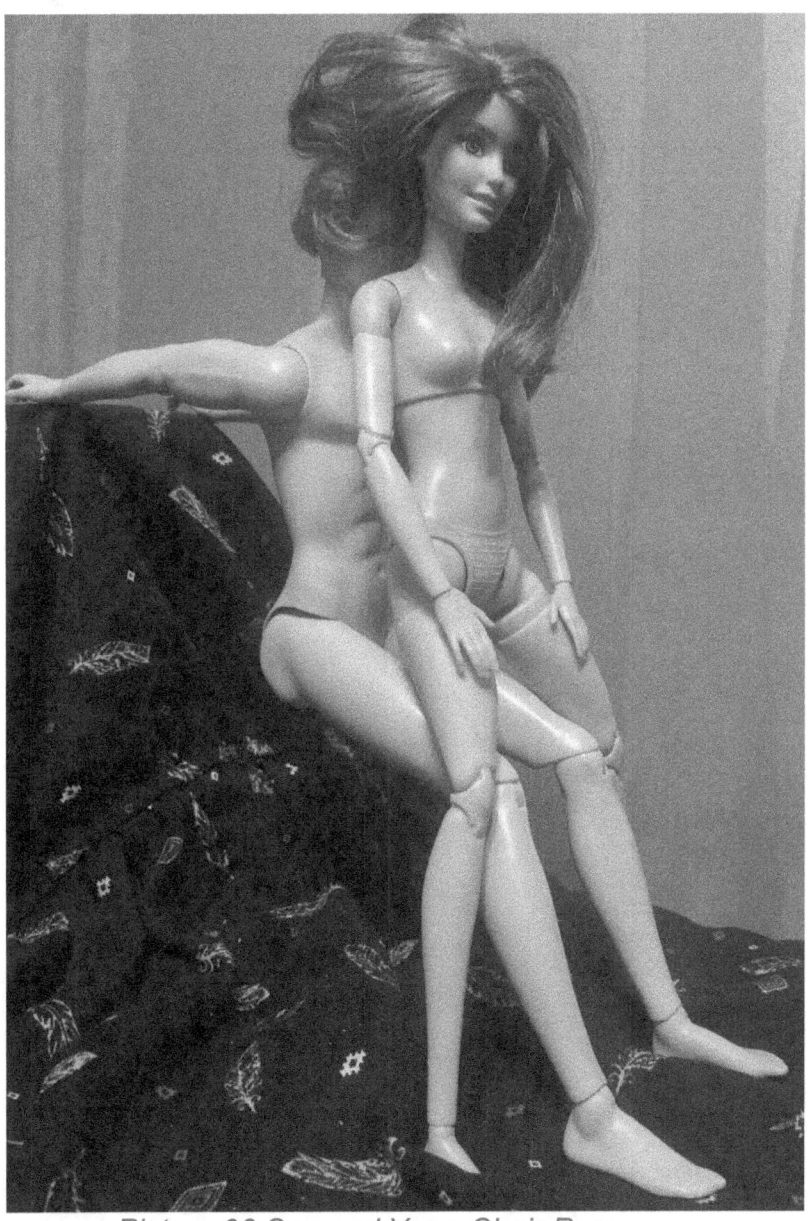

Picture 66 Sex and Yoga Chair Pose

Yoga is a great form of exercise to incorporate into your lives. Not only in sex but in an everyday workout. It also works great in combination with Tantric sex because it teaches you meditation and mindfulness. Through breathing, couples are able to be one with their own bodies and each other's. By being present in the moment, pleasurable sensations are increased enormously. Yoga is also great for loosening up the body and allowing you to explore a wide range of positions that offer different sensations for the both of you. Combine this with the art of Tantric sex and you're sure to have an intimate and explosive sexual experience!

Chapter 13: Sex Games

Because men and women are different, often times in sexual relationships the difference in sexual frequencies creates a rift between partners. There's a struggle for dominance in and outside the bedroom that leads to more fighting and less sex. But fear not! There is a solution. Sex games. They are fun and really help steam things up in the bedroom. But they also work to equalize the role of dominance between two people. Sex games also work to help cure any troubles both of you might be having in the bedroom. For instance, maybe your man is a premature ejaculator while you have trouble getting turned on in the first place. We've listed some sex games that you and your partner can play to heat things up in the bedroom. Many of these games incorporate toys that can be found in Chapter 3.

Ticking Bomb

This game is great for starting and focusing on foreplay. Often times, because men get turned on quickly, women end up not having enough foreplay which then diminishes the pleasure they get during sex. You will need a timer for this game. Start by picking a time interval, like 30 min. Set your timer to that and start it. During this time, you can touch each other, kiss, tease, or engage in whatever form of foreplay you want. The only thing you can't do is penetration. When the time is up, then you can proceed to having sexual intercourse. Foreplay is supposed to be fun. It's what stimulates both of you so that you can have amazing sex. Each time you play this game try choosing a bigger time interval. This way you can focus on giving each other pleasure and you can experiment with different types of foreplay.

Blind Man

For this game you're going to need a blindfold or something that will completely cover your partner's eyes. Start by blindfolding your partner and make sure their eyes are completely covered so that they can't see anything. Put them in the position that you want them. For instance, they can be standing, sitting or lying on the bed. Then begin by removing your hands from their body for a few moments. This will increase their anticipation and make them even more sensitive. Slowly start by lightly touching them all over. When their senses are heightened to your touch begin touching them more intensely. Focus on their sensitive areas, such as the nipples or thighs. Avoid touching their genitals until the very end. This game is good for increasing sensitivity but also for building trust. By giving up your vision you are telling your partner that you believe you are safe in their hands.

Prisoner

The Prisoner requires four lines of rope or some material that can be used as a restraint. Have your partner lay on the bed with their arms spread over their head and their legs spread apart. Tie the restraint around each of their limbs and then secure the other end of the restraint around the bed posts or something that is stable. Begin by slowly touching your partner and increasing your intensity over time. This game really allows the free partner complete control over the other's body. If you are planning on using any extreme BDSM with this game, make sure you have a safe word. For the person restrained, this game really heightens the senses and allows you to fully feel all sensations because you are powerless. This is also the same for the person who is free; it gives them an erotic sense of pleasure to be able to do whatever they want with their partner. You can also play this game in conjunction with Blind Man for a more intense experience.

Bad Girl

Bad Girl requires no equipment but if you wish you can use a paddle, a riding crop or a whip. Start by telling your man you did something bad. Give some examples to make the scenario seem more real. For an added effect, tell him you need to be punished. Then kneel on the bed or lay across his legs and let him spank you with his hand or with the chosen toy. Spanking is a great way to release any actual tension or anger either of you is feeling. As a variation you can also spank you man across the face, but make sure you've talked about it and he's ok with it. For the person being spanked, the tingly sensation received is actually quite pleasurable. It also makes your body more alert to any sensations that are happening.

Tip: Try alternation between punishment and reward. For example, spank your woman a couple times and then fondle her breasts gently. Then return with a couple more spanks, either on her buttocks or on her breasts. Continue doing this until you reach her vagina. Give her a reward by playing with it and then counter that with a few light slaps on her clitoris. This is sure to drive her wild!

War

This game is very lighthearted and actually quite fun. It requires no equipment, except for possibly a pillow (if you choose). To start, you simply have to engage in some type of "war." This could be a tickle war, a pillow fight, wrestling or any other game where you have to verse each other. The first person to surrender has to preform a sexual act for the winner. Another variation is to start with all your clothes on and whoever surrenders first has to take off a piece of clothing. You play until you're both naked. This game is great for warming both of you up and starting sex off in a lighthearted manner. It's also a great way to create some new memories that will help you associate intercourse with fun times in your relationship. Many times sexual relationships can go a bit stale but by adding something new and fun you can break out of your routines and open yourself up to experimenting with new things.

Spa Day

This isn't so much a game, as a way to pleasure each other in a different way. All you'll need is a towel and some massage oil. Have one partner lay on the towel while the other climbs on top and proceeds to massage everywhere. It feels great on tired muscles and the lubricant really heats up the sensations on the skin. Slipping your hands all over each other is a great way to get really turned on. This also helps you get in tune with each other's body. By taking the time to feel it and see what makes your partner feel good, you're learning more about them. It's a good "game" to play when you need to slow things down and reconnect. You can also play this game in combination with The Ticking Bomb and Blind Man. Enhance the ambiance by taking a bath together first and lighting some candles. Or turn it into a day where you simply focus on each other.

Sexy Cards

For this game you'll need a standard deck of cards. Start by giving each suit a meaning. For example, hearts mean touching, diamonds mean kissing and so on. The number on the card then represents the number of seconds (or minutes, if you prefer) that you perform the act for. You each take turns picking a card and doing sexy acts for each other. For example, the woman draws a 10 of hearts which means she gets to touch you for 10 seconds (or minutes). Because the game is slow, it allows you to tease each other and build up anticipation. It's even better if you make a rule that there is no penetration until the deck is completely finished.

These games are all good for helping to reduce the power play and staleness in sexual relationships. Games help ease you into a more lighthearted sexual experience. Many times, sex is stale because of routine. By throwing in a little game, you already change up something about your experience. It also gives you time to explore each other's bodies rather than rushing straight into sex. There's a more equal playing field where women are allowed to try out being the dominant one during sex. This is empowering for the woman but also extremely sexy for the man.

Chapter 14: Pornography

Pornography is generally thought of as something you watch by yourself and masturbate to. It's also commonly thought that men watch the most porn while women watch very little or not at all. This is not true. Many women and even couples watch porn to help heat up their sex life. Although there are many extreme categories of porn out there, the genre itself is not as tainted as many seem to believe.

Porn is a great way for couples, in stale sexual relationships, to learn different ways to pleasure their partner. There are many different ways to have sex and most, if not all of them, are shown in porn. If you think you and your partner could use a change in the bedroom, try watching some porn and then incorporate what you see into your sex lives. Porn has a lot of different categories that range from the more traditional to the very extreme. We've listed some of the most common categories to help you get started on what to watch.

Remember that you and your partner are sharing in this experience together. Listen to each other's tastes and try watching something that interests them but might not necessarily interest you. The point of watching porn together, is to learn about each other's fantasies and possibly act them out yourselves. Also keep in mind that the people in porn are professionals. They have been doing these things for a while so don't expect yourself or your partner to be able to perform in the same way.

- **Squirt:** This category involves men pleasuring women until they orgasm and squirt all over. For those of you that are trying to get your woman to squirt or are trying to squirt yourself, this is a good porn to watch. Not only is it extremely hot, but you get to see how it's down and what it looks like. Try incorporating some of the acting to help stimulate your own experience.

- **MILF:** MILF stands for "Mother I'd Like to Fuck" and that's exactly what these pornos are all about. The scene is usually of a boy who has sex with his friend's "hot mom". This porn is mostly geared towards men but it is also great for women around the age of being a mom. The great thing about this porn is that it shows women how sexy they can be no matter their age.

- **Amateur:** Amateur porn is when people at home make their own videos and send it to porn sites. Anyone can do this and it's becoming a bigger trend. My times, scripted porn is too unrealistic or too monotonous. Amateur porn shows people that anyone can have amazing sex like a porn star. They also tend to do things that everyday people might do in their sex lives. If you and your partner are open to it, you can also make your own porn. You can send it to porn sites or you can simply keep it for yourselves. It can get you more turned on, watching yourselves doing some erotic things in the bedroom.

- **Lesbian/Gay:** This category is mainly for the opposite sex. Men tend to get turned on by watching two girls engage in sexual activity while the opposite is true for women. Try watching both types of pornos. Sometimes it may even turn you on a little. But, if not, know that it's doing something for your partner. This porn can also help people visualize some other fantasies, such as a threesome.

- **BDSM:** As talked about in Chapter 3, pornos also have a category from BDSM. These videos can range from tame things, like restraint, to the more extreme of rape. If you are new to watching porn, it's best that you start with the simpler things first and work your way up. These pornos are good to watch if you're interested in BDSM and need somewhere to start. You can see how certain toys are used and even the way to act during a dominant/submissive session. Remember that the actors know how to use certain toys so you shouldn't immediately start using a whip, for instance, without proper instruction. This category also incorporates different types of role play that you and your partner can act out in the bedroom.

- **Public:** The public category features couples having sex in public places. This is a great porno if you've ever been fantasizing of have sex in public. You'll get to watch it happen and see how they do it. You'll probably have to be more discreet than them but you can also learn of some good places to do it. It's also great to watch if you've had sex in public before. You can try having sex in a more public place to increase the risk factor and heighten the sexual experience.

- **Rough Sex:** Rough sex is like BDSM but without the equipment. Like it's title suggests the actions performed during this are very aggressive. Many times it involves the man dominating the woman but there are other versions as well. If you've ever thought about changing up your sexual routine, this porn is for you. It shows you how to take charge and just how sexy being rough with each other can be. It will probably turn you on just watching it and all it really takes to get it started in your own bedroom is a pull of the hair or a slap.

You can use porn as a way to learn new things about sex or simply as a well to get heated up. Many times couples watch porn together because it gets them turned on and helps increase the pleasure felt during sex. There are others that use porn to learn how to change up their sexual routine. No matter what your reason is, porn is there for your use. It's considered a taboo subject but it has helped many people get out of a sexual rut and it also helps others experience different sexual sensations. There is a danger of getting addicted to porn. Make sure that you take some time to experience sex with other people rather than just with yourself. Too much porn can cause you to become desensitized to "regular" sex. It makes it harder for you to have an orgasm from sexual intercourse. You begin to need the stimulation of extreme porn to gain any pleasure from orgasm. To avoid this, only watch porn occasionally and make sure you have sexual experiences with your partner or other people. Aside from that, porn is a great outlet to learn and grow in your sexual experiences.

These are some of the more well known categories, but there are many different types of pornos out there. They can be used for self-pleasure or as a learning tool for couples. There are many couples out there that also watch porn together for the simple pleasure. It can get you hot imagining each other in those porn scenarios and it can give you new ideas to experiment with. However, porn isn't for everyone. Don't force your partner to watch something if it makes them uncomfortable. Talk about the idea first and if they seem on the fence, suggest something mild, like Amateur porn. If they enjoy it you can start proposing other categories. Try to get them to open up and suggest something they might want to see. By doing this, you get to open up to each other and share some of your deeper fantasies. Often times, couples bury their fantasies because they think it's not right or makes them weird. By watching porn, you learn that, just about every fantasy is out there and has been experienced by someone. It helps you open up and realize that your fantasies don't make you strange.

Chapter 15: Anal Sex

There are many opposing thoughts when it comes to anal sex. Many women say they've tried it and they love it while others are completely against even mentioning it. Chances are your partner has brought it up once or twice and maybe you've been thinking about it. Well we're here to tell you that, you should go for it. Although, it may seem painful it can actually be quite enjoyable. If you've decided to try it here are some tips to help ease yourself into the experience.

- Don't try it if you really don't want to. If you're just doing it to make your partner happy, then you shouldn't do it. The anus is very different from the vagina and so it must be treated differently. The sensations felt are also very different. If you want this to be easier make sure that it's something you really want to do. This will make you more confident and help you relax.

- Use a condom. You may think that because it's your anus, you won't get pregnant but that isn't true. Semen that drips out of your anus could come into contact with your vagina and cause a pregnancy. A condom is also good for keeping bacteria from spreading anywhere. Never use the same condom for anal and vaginal sex.

- Use lots of lube. The anus doesn't natural produce any lubrication so you are going to have to use lube to reduce the amount of friction caused by thrusting. It also helps the penis slip in easier.

- Warm up. The anus goes pretty much unused, except for releasing excrement, so it's very tight. If you try to put a penis in there right away it will hurt and it could cause your anus to tear. To avoid this, make sure you take time to warm up. This means your partner should start by fingering you with one finger and working his way up. You can also buy a butt plug to help loosen you up. The butt plug is tapered so when it's inside of you it won't slip out. This means you can insert it and then proceed with vaginal sex. Your anus will get use to the feeling of having something inside it, plus it's an added sensation that makes an orgasm more intense.

- Relax. When you're ready to have your partner insert his penis, try to relax as much as possible. This will make it hurt less and help the penis go in easier. The tip is what hurts the most because it's the widest part of the penis. Once you get past that it should feel a little better. Make sure your partner goes slow. He could cause injury if he goes too fast.

- You're going to feel like you're pooping. The most uncomfortable thing about this pose is that you feel like you're pooping. Chances are you're probably not and you probably won't. If this is something you're really worried about, do this pose after you've gone to the bathroom. This way you know you've emptied everything out. You can also lie a towel down for easy clean up, just in case a little poop comes out.

- Have your partner stimulate other parts of your body. Anal stimulation usually isn't enough to get a woman to orgasm. Your partner can play with your nipples, vagina, clitoris, etc. to help you reach orgasm. This should only be done when you are more comfortable with anal. While you are still new to this you should focus on experiencing the thrusting movement.

- Doggy style is the best position to start off in. This position puts your anus at the most comfortable height and angle for the penis to enter. The easier it is to put in, the better it will feel. You're also able to relax your anal muscles more while you're in this position.

Anal sex is a great way to intensify your sex life. It's a very taboo sexual experience which makes it all the more exciting to try out. If you're trying it for the first time, remember that you need to take control. This is a completely new sensation for women so you need to control what your partner is doing. For him, it only feels more tight. He doesn't know if he's hurting you or not. Guide him in and tell him when you want him to stop. Anal sex can be a very pleasurable experience if you enter into it slowly.

When you get more experienced with anal you can start adding more things to it. You can use toys or experiment with different role plays. It's also highly enjoyable if you start with vaginal sex and end with anal. Just make sure you don't go the other way around. Once your anus is use to the sensations your partner will be able to thrust much harder and faster. This is really great for those that enjoy rougher sex. Anal sex, like vaginal sex, feels wonderful for both partners and really allows you to explore the full range of sexual experiences offered to you. It can also be combined with Tantric sex for a deeper connection that requires a lot of trust.

Chapter 16: Defloration

Defloration, also known as "popping the cherry," is a term used to describe taking someone's virginity. This is a very big deal, for both men and women. Men usually want to loose their virginity as quickly as possible, while women want to wait for that special moment. Whatever the case, taking someone's virginity is a big deal, physically and emotionally.

If both partners are virgins, this often makes things a little easier. There's no pressure to perform amazingly. However, there are times when one partner is more experienced than the other. When this happens, the more experienced partner needs to take charge. If you are not as experienced, listen to them but also talk about what your feeling. They've been in the same position before and can often help ease your worries. Communication and trust are a big thing when it comes to defloration. This is a big step for both partners. It should be safe, pleasurable and fun.

Women

Women are usually told that losing their virginity is one of the biggest steps in their life and for some it is. However, this doesn't go for everyone. It is true that you should wait to lose it with someone you trust and are comfortable with but there isn't really a perfect moment. If you feel you are ready to lose your virginity, here are some things you should keep in mind.

- Relax. Losing your virginity can cause all sorts of anxious thoughts to arise, which makes your body tense and can cause you to have a bad first experience. Try reading up on what happens during sex. By understanding your body and your partner's, you have some idea of what's going to happen.
- Be positive. When you choose to lose your virginity is your choice. Don't let society tell you that you have to wait to get married or that you're a bad person if you do it too early. But at the same time, don't let anyone pressure you into having sex. It's supposed to be something that brings you

and your partner closer together. Don't let anyone try to shame your new experience.

- Prepare. When you and your partner decide you're ready to have sex, make sure you have all the necessary equipment. Go to the store and buy some condoms and lubricant. Condoms will help protect you from STI's (sexually-transmitted infections) and from getting pregnant. Lubricant will help reduce friction which will ease most of the pain. The best lubricant for your first time is a silicon or water based lube. It's very slippery plus it doesn't harm the integrity of the condom.

- Talk to your partner. If you're feeling nervous or even excited, let your partner know. They're probably thinking the same thing. It's good to share these emotions and/or concerns with each other before having sex. It helps both of you reassure each other that you're there for one another.

- You may bleed. The hymen is a thin membrane that's covering part of the vaginal opening. If you hold a mirror down to you vagina you should see it. Usually it starts to wear away because of different activities such as playing sports, riding horses or using tampons. If you're younger your hymen is probably still intact, which means that when penetration occurs it will stretch and break. However, this doesn't happen all the time. Sometimes it just stretches without breaking. If it does break there will normally be a little bit of blood. Usually only a light bit of spotting for a few hours. The good thing is, it doesn't hurt. If you do experience pain during sex it's probably caused by the friction from thrusting. The more relaxed you are the less pain there will be.

- Take your time. Don't' rush into having sex right away. Start out with lots of foreplay. This will give you time to relax and will also help get you more warmed up. Make sure you communicate with your partner. If at any time you want to stop, let them know. Losing your virginity can be a scary thing, so don't feel that you need to rush into it. If the moment isn't right, then you can always try another time.

Men

Men are generally different when it comes to losing their virginity. Often times they are encouraged to get rid of it as soon as possible. It's seen as the threshold to going from being a boy to a man. But losing their virginity is also a big step in life. Teaching boys the right way to have sex not only improves their sex life, it helps them learn how to make their woman feel amazing.

- Relax. For men, it's usually a race to lose their virginity. Sometimes, they often have sex with a random girl, simply to become a man. But this shouldn't be the case. Wait to have sex with someone you really care about. Society may tell you that you're not a man if you haven't had sex, but that isn't true. Waiting for the right person, who you love and respect is what really makes you a man.
- Don't overthink. Men tend to worry that the first time they have sex they'll be bad at it. This is true, but don't let it get to you. This is the first time you're going to have sex. No one expects you to have the best moves. Don't try to do anything fancy because you'll probably end up looking foolish. You'll have plenty of chances to practice your moves.
- Have the right stuff. If you and your partner decide that it's time to lose your virginity, make sure you're prepared with condoms and lube. The condoms will help protect you from getting any STI's (sexually-transmitted infections) and the lube will help make your partner more wet which will reduce the friction. Friction is good for men but sometimes if it's too much, it can pull at the skin and cause discomfort of even a rash. Your penis is going to be very sensitive once it orgasms, so you want to minimize any risk of injury.
- Read up. Learning about your partner's anatomy may help make it less nerve-wracking when it comes time for you to have sex. By knowing where everything is you have a much better chance of it looking like you know what you're doing. It also helps if you familiarize yourself with the vaginal opening. Many times men think it's a lot higher than it is. By

locating the vaginal opening right away, you make penetration a lot smoother.

• Be gentle. If your partner is also a virgin take it slow. There's no need to pull any fancy moves that could cause her discomfort. As much as you want to "put it in her" it's also important to remember that she is warmed up enough. Girls' need more foreplay than men, especially if she is a virgin. She's probably just as nervous as you at performing adequately and will need you to comfort her and ease her into it.

• Communicate. Men are notoriously bad at telling people their feelings. But in this case it would be a good idea to share what you're feeling with your partner. Chances are she's just as nervous as you. By letting her know you feel the same way, you can reassure yourself and help make her less nervous.

• Focus on foreplay. As much as you want to jump quickly to intercourse, make sure you spend enough time on foreplay. This will make the experience feel much better for both of you. Even if you don't know what you're doing, try going down on her. This will help her lubricate which will reduce the friction. Insert one finger and then two (if possible) into her vagina. Slowly thrust them in and out, mimicking penis movement. This will stretch out the vagina and make it easier for your penis to go in.

@ Copyright 2017. All rights reserved.

All rights Reserved. No part of this publication or the information in it may be quoted from or reproduced in any form by means such as printing, scanning, photocopying or otherwise without prior written permission of the copyright holder.

Disclaimer and Terms of Use: Effort has been made to ensure that the information in this book is accurate and complete, however, the author and the publisher do not warrant the accuracy of the information, text and graphics contained within the book due to the rapidly changing nature of science, research, known and unknown facts and internet. The Author and the publisher do not hold any responsibility for errors, omissions or contrary interpretation of the subject matter herein. This book is presented solely for motivational and informational purposes only.

www.ingramcontent.com/pod-product-compliance
Lightning Source LLC
Chambersburg PA
CBHW072136280526
45788CB00002B/665